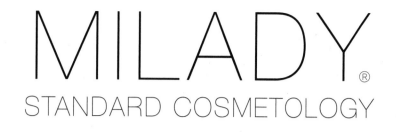

MILADY®
STANDARD COSMETOLOGY

P9-DWT-322

PRACTICAL WORKBOOK

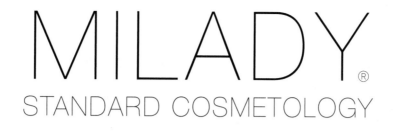

MILADY®
STANDARD COSMETOLOGY

PRACTICAL WORKBOOK

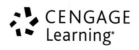

CENGAGE
Learning®

Australia • Brazil • Japan • Korea • Mexico • Singapore • Spain • United Kingdom • United States

**Milady Standard Cosmetology
Practical Workbook, 2016 Edition**

Executive Director, Milady: Sandra Bruce

Product Director: Corina Santoro

Product Manager: Philip I. Mandl

Senior Content Developer: Jessica Mahoney

Product Assistants: Harry Garrott and
Michelle Whitehead

Senior Director of Sales and Marketing:
Gerard McAvey

Marketing Manager: Elizabeth Bushey

Senior Production Director: Wendy Troeger

Production Director: Patty Stephan

Senior Content Project Manager:
Nina Tucciarelli

Senior Art Director: Benj Gleeksman

Cover image(s):

Hair by Ted Gibson
Photography by Yuki and Joseph Paradiso
Makeup Artist: Valenté Frazier

© 2016, 2012, 2008 Milady, a part of Cengage Learning

WCN: 01-100-101

ALL RIGHTS RESERVED. No part of this work covered by the copyright herein may be reproduced, transmitted, stored, or used in any form or by any means graphic, electronic, or mechanical, including but not limited to photocopying, recording, scanning, digitizing, taping, Web distribution, information networks, or information storage and retrieval systems, except as permitted under Section 107 or 108 of the 1976 United States Copyright Act, without the prior written permission of the publisher.

For product information and technology assistance, contact us at
Cengage Learning Customer & Sales Support, 1-800-354-9706

For permission to use material from this text or product,
submit all requests online at **www.cengage.com/permissions**
Further permissions questions can be e-mailed to
permissionrequest@cengage.com

Library of Congress Control Number: 2 0 1 4 9 5 0 2 7 9

ISBN: 978-1-2857-6947-9

Milady
20 Channel Center Street
Boston, MA 02210
USA

Cengage Learning is a leading provider of customized learning solutions with office locations around the globe, including Singapore, the United Kingdom, Australia, Mexico, Brazil, and Japan. Locate your local office at: **international.cengage.com/region**

Cengage Learning products are represented in Canada by Nelson Education, Ltd.

For your lifelong learning solutions, visit **www.milady.com**

Purchase any of our products at your local college store or at our preferred online store **www.cengagebrain.com**

Visit our corporate website at **cengage.com**

Notice to the Reader

Publisher does not warrant or guarantee any of the products described herein or perform any independent analysis in connection with any of the product information contained herein. Publisher does not assume, and expressly disclaims, any obligation to obtain and include information other than that provided to it by the manufacturer. The reader is expressly warned to consider and adopt all safety precautions that might be indicated by the activities described herein and to avoid all potential hazards. By following the instructions contained herein, the reader willingly assumes all risks in connection with such instructions. The publisher makes no representations or warranties of any kind, including but not limited to, the warranties of fitness for particular purpose or merchantability, nor are any such representations implied with respect to the material set forth herein, and the publisher takes no responsibility with respect to such material. The publisher shall not be liable for any special, consequential, or exemplary damages resulting, in whole or part, from the readers' use of, or reliance upon, this material.

Printed in the United States of America
Print Number: 01   Print Year: 2015

CONTENTS

INTRODUCTION

Congratulations! As a student of cosmetology, you now hold in your hands an important tool designed to help you successfully progress through your course of study. You have chosen to embark upon a career in cosmetology, and that can be a life-transforming event. In this journey, you deserve the best possible education, and that can be accomplished by using the best possible educational tools available. The *Milady Standard Cosmetology Practical Workbook* is one of those tools.

Purpose

The purpose of the *Milady Standard Cosmetology Practical Workbook* is to act as a study tool for you to achieve the objectives of each lesson presented by your instructors. Each chapter is designed to accompany the chapters you will be assigned in the *Milady Standard Cosmetology* textbook. The workbook is comprised of written questions including essay, fill-in-the-blank, true/false, multiple choice, and matching. You will also find a new addition to the true/false questions if you choose "false" as the answer. Space is provided where you will need to insert the rationale for why the answer is false. Each chapter also includes an extra activity that may require additional research or completion of a subject-related project to help reinforce your understanding of the textbook.

HOW TO USE
THIS WORKBOOK

This workbook should be used with the *Milady Standard Cosmetology* and the *Milady Standard Cosmetology Theory Workbook.* This workbook directly follows the practical information found in the student textbook. Pages to be read and studied are listed at the beginning of each chapter. Additional theoretical information and exercises can be found in the *Milady Standard Cosmetology Theory Workbook.*

The best practice is to close your textbook and see how much you have retained after reading the chapter and taking part in the classroom lessons presented by your instructor. Answer each question in this workbook with a pencil after consulting your textbook for correct information. Questions can be corrected and/or rated during class or individually. Consult with your instructor to ensure that you are using this workbook in the manner intended and to determine how credit will be awarded for your completion of the exercises contained herein.

CHAPTER 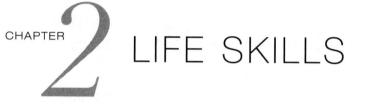 HISTORY & CAREER OPPORTUNITIES

See Milady Standard Cosmetology Theory Workbook.

CHAPTER 2 LIFE SKILLS

See Milady Standard Cosmetology Theory Workbook.

CHAPTER 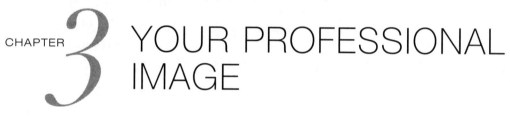 YOUR PROFESSIONAL IMAGE

See Milady Standard Cosmetology Theory Workbook.

CHAPTER 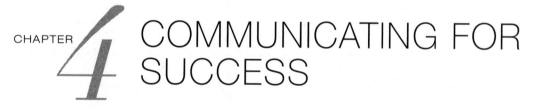 COMMUNICATING FOR SUCCESS

See Milady Standard Cosmetology Theory Workbook.

CHAPTER 5

INFECTION CONTROL: PRINCIPLES & PRACTICES

Date: _____

Rating: _____

Text Pages: 68–111

why study INFECTION CONTROL: PRINCIPLES & PRACTICES?

1. List the five reasons why it is important for cosmetologists to study and thoroughly understand infection control principles and practices.

1) _____

_____

_____

2) _____

_____

_____

3) _____

_____

_____

4) _____

_____

_____

5) _____

_____

_____

Meet the Current Regulations for Health and Safety

2. State agencies set guidelines for the manufacturing, sale, and use of equipment and chemical ingredients.

_____ True   _____ False

Rationale:

3. OSHA is part of the U.S. Department of _____.

4. The _____ created the Hazard Communication Standard (HCS), which requires that chemical manufacturers and importers assess and communicate the potential hazards associated with their products.

5. The standards set by OSHA address which of the following issues? Check all that apply.

_____ a) Handling and mixing of products

_____ b) General workplace safety

_____ c) Potentially hazardous product ingredients

_____ d) Storing and disposing of products

6. As of June 2015, both federal and state laws require that manufacturers supply a _____ for all chemical products manufactured and sold.

7. Where should you look to locate the names of hazardous ingredients used in a chemical salon product?

_____ a) The manufacturer's invoice

_____ b) The product's SDS

_____ c) The salon's employee handbook

_____ d) The Environmental Protection Agency's (EPA) website

8. The identification category of the SDS includes the recommended use of product and restrictions on use.

_____ True   _____ False

Rationale:

9. The toxicology information category of the SDS lists the chemical stability and possibility of hazardous reactions.

_____ True   _____ False

Rationale:

10. How does an employee verify that he or she has read an SDS?

_____

_____

_____

_____

11. Which of the following are destroyed by disinfectants? Check all that apply.

_____ a) Most bacteria   _____ c) Viruses on surfaces

_____ b) Fungi   _____ d) Spores

12. Is it safe to use a hospital disinfectant on a nonporous surface in the salon; why or why not?

_____

_____

_____

_____

13. An item that is made or constructed of a material with no pores or openings and that cannot absorb liquids is considered _____.

14. When disinfecting your equipment, you should always choose a tuberculocidal disinfectant.

_____ True   _____ False

> Rationale:

15. Before a manufacturer can sell a product for disinfecting surfaces, tools, implements, or equipment, they must obtain _____ number that certifies that the disinfectant, when used correctly, will be effective against the pathogens listed on the label.

16. A state regulatory agency can issue penalties against both a salon owner and the cosmetologist's license.

_____ True   _____ False

> Rationale:

17. What levels of legislature writes laws to determine the scope of practice?

_____

18. Laws are more specific than rules and regulations.

_____ True   _____ False

> Rationale:

19. It is the responsibility of the cosmetologist to be aware of any changes or updates to the rules and regulations that apply to their work in the salon and to comply with them.

_____ True   _____ False

Rationale:

Understand the Principles of Infection

20. If your actions result in an injury or infection, you could lose your license.

_____ True   _____ False

Rationale:

21. An _____ disease may be spread from one person to another person.

_____ True   _____ False

Rationale:

22. What is it called when you scrub something with soap and water or detergent and water to remove all visible dirt, debris, and many disease-causing germs.

_____ a) Cleaning   _____ c) Sterilizing

_____ b) Disinfecting   _____ d) Sanitizing

23. Disinfection destroys all organisms on surfaces.

_____ True   _____ False

Rationale:

24. Which of the following disinfectants are used in salons? Check all that apply.

_____ a) Fungicidal   _____ c) Virucidal

_____ b) Sporicidal   _____ d) Bactericidal

25. When mixing and using a disinfectant, you must always follow the instructions on the label to ensure that it is used safely and effectively.

_____ True   _____ False

Rationale:

26. Contaminated salon tools and equipment can spread infections from client to client if the proper _____ steps are not taken after every service.

27. Where can bacteria exist?

_____

_____

_____

28. A surface is considered free of bacteria as long as it looks clean to the naked eye.

_____ True   _____ False

Rationale:

29. Differentiate between the two primary types of bacteria.

_____

_____

_____

_____

_____

_____

30. Which type of bacteria causes pneumonia?

      _____ a) Bacilli   _____ c) Diplococci

      _____ b) Staphylococci   _____ d) Streptococci

31. Staphylococci:

      _____ a) are not pus-forming.

      _____ b) grow in clusters like bunches of grapes.

      _____ c) cause strep throat and blood poisoning.

      _____ d) cause tetanus and typhoid fever.

32. Which type of bacteria causes Lyme disease?

      _____ a) Bacilli   _____ c) Spirilla

      _____ b) Staphylococci   _____ d) Diplococci

33. All cocci use slender, hairlike extensions called flagella for locomotion.

      _____ True   _____ False

Rationale:

34. Identify the three ways in which cocci are generally transmitted.

    1) _____

    2) _____

    3) _____

35. Some bacteria and viruses can produce toxins.

      _____ True   _____ False

Rationale:

36. Bacteria multiply best in cool, bright, dry places.

_____ True   _____ False

```
Rationale:



```

37. During the _____ or _____ stage, certain bacteria can coat themselves with wax-like outer shells during infavorable conditions.

38. What are the four signs of inflammation?

1) _____

2) _____

3) _____

4) _____

39. An abscess is an example of a _____.

40. Staphylococci are a relatively rare form of bacteria that can affect humans.

_____ True   _____ False

```
Rationale:



```

41. Staph bacteria can be picked up on doorknobs, countertops, and other surfaces, but in the salon they are more frequently spread through skin-to-skin contact.

_____ True   _____ False

```
Rationale:



```

42. How does methicillin-resistant Staphylococcus aureus (MRSA) commonly manifest and evolve (if left untreated)?

_____

_____

_____

43. A virus can replicate only by taking over the host cell's reproductive function.

_____ True   _____ False

Rationale:

44. Viral infections can be treated with antibiotics.

_____ True   _____ False

Rationale:

45. It is strongly recommended that cosmetologists be vaccinated for which strain of hepatitis?

_____ a) Hepatitis A   _____ c) Hepatitis C

_____ b) Hepatitis B   _____ d) Hepatitis D

46. A(n) _____ is a reaction due to extreme sensitivity to certain foods, chemicals, or other normally harmless substances.

47. Lice and mites cause what type of disease?

_____ a) Pathogenic   _____ c) Systemic

_____ b) Parasitic   _____ d) Viral

48. Which of the following is a sign of human papilloma virus (HPV) infection?

_____ a) Small black dots on the bottom of the foot

_____ b) Redness and swelling around a healing wound

_____ c) Yellowing of the eyes

_____ d) Yellowing of the toenails

49. Cosmetologists cannot cut live skin, but they are authorized to remove calluses.

_____ True   _____ False

Rationale:

50. In general, it is easy to contract hepatitis.

_____ True   _____ False

Rationale:

51. Explain how HIV spreads.

_____

_____

_____

_____

_____

52. If you accidentally cut a client who is HIV-positive, the multiuse tool must be discarded and never used again.

_____ True   _____ False

Rationale:

53. Mildew is a common cause of human infections in the salon.

_____ True   _____ False

Rationale:

54. The technical term for barbers itch is _____.

55. It is recommended that you use _____ to quickly remove visible hair and debris from clippers.

56. Discuss how nail infections are spread.

_____

_____

_____

57. Tinea pedis is a _____ fungus of the foot.

58. Head lice are a type of parasite responsible for contagious diseases and conditions.

_____ True   _____ False

Rationale:

59. Contagious diseases and conditions caused by parasites should only be treated by a doctor.

_____ True   _____ False

Rationale:

60. _____ immunity is partly inherited and partly developed through healthy living, while _____ immunity is immunity that the body develops after overcoming a disease, through inoculation, or through exposure to natural allergens.

Prevent the Spread of Disease

61. Proper infection control requires two steps:

_____

_____

_____

62. Identify and describe the accepted method for testing an autoclave.

_____

_____

63. List three ways to clean tools or implements.

1) _____

_____

2) _____

_____

3) _____

_____

64. Using disinfectants as hand cleaners can cause skin irritation and _____.

65. When mixing a disinfectant concentrate and water, you:

_____ a) pour the water and disinfectant concentrate into a third container simultaneously.

_____ b) always add the water to the disinfectant concentrate.

_____ c) always add the disinfectant concentrate to the water.

_____ d) can combine the two substances in any order you choose.

66. All disinfectants have the same concentration.

_____ True   _____ False

Rationale:

67. _____, when applied to disinfectant claims, means the effectiveness with which a disinfecting solution kills microorganisms when used according to the label instructions.

68. All tools and implements can be disinfected.

_____ True   _____ False

Rationale:

69. Why must all implements be thoroughly cleaned of all visible matter or residue before being placed in disinfectant solution?

_____

70. List the eight recommended tips for using disinfectants.

1) _____

_____

_____

2) _____

_____

_____

3) _____

_____

_____

4) _____

_____

_____

5) _____

_____

_____

6) _____

_____

_____

7) _____

_____

_____

8) _____

_____

_____

71. Explain what is meant by complete immersion.

_____

_____

_____

72. What are quats?

_____

_____

73. Quat solutions usually disinfect surfaces and implements in:

_____ a) 5 minutes.   _____ c) 15 minutes.

_____ b) 10 minutes.   _____ d) 20 minutes.

74. Phenolic disinfectants:

_____ a) are completely safe for the environment.

_____ b) are not tuberculocidal.

_____ c) have a very low pH.

_____ d) Are a form of formaldehyde.

75. Phenolic disinfectants have a low pH and are safe on the skin.

_____ True   _____ False

Rationale:

76. The technical term for household bleach is _____.

77. A fresh bleach solution should be mixed every 24 hours or when the solution has been contaminated.

_____ True   _____ False

Rationale:

78. Explain how to mix and maintain a bleach solution.

_____

_____

_____

_____

_____

_____

79. List the safety tips for using disinfectants.

a) _____

_____

b) _____

_____

c) _____

_____

d) _____

_____

e) _____

_____

f) _____

_____

g) _____

_____

h) _____

_____

i) _____

_____

80. What are the two things you should never do when using disinfectants?

1) _____

_____

2) _____

_____

81. Multiuse items must have hard, nonporous surfaces.

_____ True   _____ False

Rationale:

82. Single-use items cannot be properly cleaned so that all visible residue is removed.

_____ True   _____ False

Rationale:

83. What are three examples of multiuse tools?

_____

_____

84. Define the term porous.

_____

_____

85. Some porous items can be safely cleaned, disinfected, and used again.

_____ True   _____ False

Rationale:

86. Single-use items must be thrown out after each use.

_____ True   _____ False

Rationale:

87. List eight examples of single-use items.

1) _____

2) _____

3) _____

4) _____

5) _____

6) _____

7) _____

8) _____

88. Salons should keep a logbook as required by certain state boards for inspections and to provide clients peace of mind and confidence in the cosmetologist's ability to protect the client from infection and disease. What types of information should the logbook contain?

a) _____

b) _____

c) _____

d) _____

e) _____

89. List the eight steps involved in disinfecting nonelectrical tools and implements.

1) _____

_____

_____

2) _____

_____

_____

3) _____

_____

_____

4) _____

_____

_____

5) _____

_____

_____

6) _____

_____

_____

7) _____

_____

_____

8) _____

_____

_____

90. Explain how to clean and disinfect electrical equipment.

_____

_____

_____

_____

_____

91. Why is it important to ensure towels, linens, and capes are thoroughly dried?

_____

92. To prevent capes used for cutting, shampooing, and chemical services from touching a client's skin, use _____.

93. List the procedure for cleaning and disinfecting whirlpool, air-jet, and pipeless foot spas after each client.

a) _____

_____

_____

_____

b) _____

_____

_____

_____

c) _____

_____

_____

_____

d) _____

_____

_____

_____

e) _____

_____

_____

_____

f) _____

_____

_____

_____

g) _____

_____

_____

_____

h) _____

_____

_____

_____

i) _____

_____

_____

_____

j) _____

_____

_____

_____

k) _____

_____

_____

_____

l) _____

_____

_____

_____

m) _____

_____

_____

_____

94. List the steps to clean and disinfect basic foot basins or tubs.

a) _____

b) _____

_____

c) _____

d) _____

_____

_____

_____

_____

_____

e) _____

f) _____

_____

95. Discuss the action and use of chelating soaps.

_____

_____

_____

_____

_____

96. Additives, powders, and tablets can eliminate the need to clean and disinfect.

_____ True   _____ False

Rationale:

97. _____ is one of the most important actions you can take to prevent germs from spreading from one person to another.

98. Medical studies suggest that antimicrobial and antibacterial soaps are no more effective than regular soaps and detergents.

_____ True   _____ False

Rationale:

99. What is the procedure for proper hand washing?

a) _____

_____

_____

_____

_____

b) _____

_____

_____

_____

_____

c) _____

_____

_____

_____

_____

d) _____

_____

_____

_____

100. Partner with another student and write a song (catchphrase, rap, or poem) about the correct hand washing procedure or methods for preventing the spread of germs. Consider the timing to ensure that proper hand washing can be completed in the same time it takes to recite the lyrics. Write the verses in the space provided below.

_____

_____

_____

_____

_____

_____

_____

_____

_____

_____

Follow Standard Precautions to Protect you and your Clients

101. The term _____ refers to guidelines published by the Centers for Disease Control and Prevention (CDC) that require employers and employees to assume that all human blood and body fluids are potentially infectious.

102. Define the term *asymptomatic*.

_____

_____

103. What are the three main precautions that protect salon employees in situations in which they could be exposed to blood-borne pathogens?

1) _____

_____

2) _____

_____

3) _____

_____

104. Explain the proper procedure for removing gloves.

_____

_____

_____

_____

_____

_____

105. Contact with nonintact (broken) skin, blood, body fluid, or other potentially infectious materials as a result of the performance of an employee's duties is known as a(n):

_____ a) infectious disease.   _____ c) exposure incident.

_____ b) decontamination.   _____ d) inflammation.

106. If you suffer a cut or an abrasion that bleeds during a service, what should you do?

a) _____

_____

_____

_____

b) _____

_____

_____

_____

c) _____

_____

_____

_____

d) _____

_____

_____

_____

e) _____

_____

_____

_____

_____

f) _____

_____

_____

g) _____

_____

_____

_____

_____

List your Professional Responsibilities

107. List the 21 recommended guidelines for keeping a salon looking its best. We will provide a few answers to get you started.

1) Keep floors and workstations dust-free. Sweep hair off the floor after every client. Mop floors and vacuum carpets every day.

2) _____

_____

3) _____

_____

4) _____

_____

5) _____

_____

6) _____

_____

7) _____

_____

8) _____

_____

9) _____

_____

10) _____

_____

11) _____

_____

12) _____

_____

13) _____

_____

14) _____

_____

15) _____

_____

16) _____

_____

17) _____

_____

18) _____

_____

19) _____

_____

20) _____

_____

_____

21) _____

_____

108. ☻ **ACTIVITY**: Consider and compare safety practices in the home and in the salon.

Observe and list the various safety steps you take each day in your home. For example, do you properly store cords for blow dryers or curling irons after use to ensure no one trips over them? Do you always check to make sure electrical appliances are turned off when not in use? Do you always wash your hands thoroughly before preparing food, and so forth?

Also observe and list any incorrect safety procedures practiced by you or other family members. For example, is a stove burner left on? Do family members "double dip" when eating certain foods, and so forth?

After creating your lists, write a brief narrative below comparing how the practices you observed compare to safe practices in the salon.

_____

_____

_____

CHAPTER **6** # GENERAL ANATOMY & PHYSIOLOGY

See Milady Standard Cosmetology Theory Workbook.

CHAPTER **7** # SKIN STRUCTURE, GROWTH, & NUTRITION

See Milady Standard Cosmetology Theory Workbook.

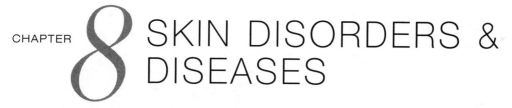

CHAPTER **8** # SKIN DISORDERS & DISEASES

See Milady Standard Cosmetology Theory Workbook.

CHAPTER **9** # NAIL STRUCTURE & GROWTH

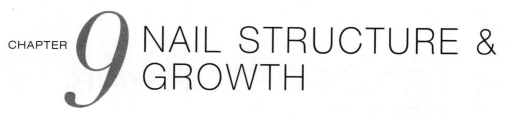

See Milady Standard Cosmetology Theory Workbook.

CHAPTER 10 NAIL DISORDERS & DISEASES

See Milady Standard Cosmetology Theory Workbook.

CHAPTER 11 PROPERTIES OF THE HAIR & SCALP

See Milady Standard Cosmetology Theory Workbook.

CHAPTER 12 BASICS OF CHEMISTRY

See Milady Standard Cosmetology Theory Workbook.

CHAPTER 13 BASICS OF ELECTRICITY

See Milady Standard Cosmetology Theory Workbook.

CHAPTER 14 PRINCIPLES OF HAIR DESIGN

See Milady Standard Cosmetology Theory Workbook.

CHAPTER 15 SCALP CARE, SHAMPOOING, & CONDITIONING

Date: _____

Rating: _____

Text Pages: 320–355

1. The shampoo is one of the most important experiences a stylist provides.

    _____ True   _____ False

    > Rationale:
    >
    >
    >
    >

2. What are the three different processes of the shampoo service?

    1) _____

    2) _____

    3) _____

why study SCALP CARE, SHAMPOOING, AND CONDITIONING?

3. In your own words, explain why cosmetologists should study and thoroughly understand scalp care, shampooing, and conditioning.

    _____

    _____

    _____

    _____

    _____

    _____

Safely and Effectively Use Massage in Scalp Care

4. The two basic requirements for a healthy scalp are _____ and
   _____.

5. Usually done once the hair has been cleansed, _____ are initiated
   along with the conditioning service.

6. Proper maintenance of the hair and scalp begins with the hygiene practice of
   shampooing.

   _____ True   _____ False

Rationale:

7. The difference between a relaxation massage and a treatment massage are the
   products used.

   _____ True   _____ False

Rationale:

8. Treatment massages are generally suggested to address conditions of the scalp such
   as dryness, minimal flaking, and to temporarily _____.

9. Scalp massage is not appropriate for clients with which of the following?

   _____ a) Circulatory condition   _____ c) High blood pressure

   _____ b) Severe, uncontrolled hypertension   _____ d) Diabetes

10. Cosmetologists who talk during scalp massage enhance the procedure's relaxation
    therapy.

    _____ True   _____ False

Rationale:

11. Explain how to commence the scalp massage procedure.

_____

_____

_____

12. Discuss the purpose of a general scalp treatment and when it should be recommended.

_____

_____

_____

13. When should a dry hair and scalp treatment be used?

_____

_____

_____

14. Outline the special requirements and implements of a dry hair and scalp treatment.

_____

_____

_____

_____

15. During a dry hair and scalp treatment, a scalp steamer can be applied to _____ in the hair.

16. Excessive oiliness is caused by _____.

17. Sebaceous glands are sometimes active due to _____ but can also be aggravated by _____, misuse and layering of heavy products, and physical changes in the body.

18. _____ is the result of a fungus called malassezia.

19. The use of _____ used with massage could help to penetrate the product into the hair shaft and scalp while keeping the scalp _____ enough to loosen and lift the agitated cells that should be removed from the scalp during the rinse and potentially after the shampoo.

Learn the Benefits of Proper Hair Brushing

20. What are the benefits of correct hair brushing?

_____

_____

21. When should a stylist avoid brushing hair?

    a) _____

    b) _____

    c) _____

    d) _____

22. The most highly recommended hairbrushes are made from _____ bristles.

23. Hairbrushes with _____ bristles are shiny and smooth and are more suitable for hairstyling.

24. List the steps in the hair brushing procedure. The first and last steps have been filled in for you to help you get started.

    a) Show your client to the shampoo chair and assist him or her in becoming comfortable.

    b) _____

    _____

    _____

    c) _____

    _____

    _____

    d) _____

    _____

    _____

    e) _____

    _____

    _____

f) _____

_____

_____

g) _____

_____

_____

h) _____

_____

_____

i) _____

_____

_____

j) _____

_____

_____

k) _____

_____

_____

l) Now move on to the next portion of the service.

Provide a Proper and Effective Shampoo Service

25. Always check the scalp and hair for any of the following conditions that may alter your product choices or even your professional ability to perform the service:

a) _____

b) _____

c) _____

d) _____

e) _____

f) _____

g) _____

h) _____

i) _____

26. The cosmetologist can massage or manipulate a client's scalp when reddened scalp irritations are present.

_____ True   _____ False

Rationale:

27. Hair should only be shampooed as often as necessary.

_____ True   _____ False

Rationale:

28. Excessive shampooing strips the hair of its protective oil, called _____, that, in small amounts, seals and protects the hair's cuticle.

29. As a general rule, oily hair must be shampooed less often than normal or dry hair.

_____ True   _____ False

Rationale:

30. List the steps in the basic shampooing and conditioning procedure. Since this is a long list of steps, some steps have been filled in to help you.

a) Show your client to the shampoo chair and assist him or her in becoming comfortable.

b) _____

_____

_____

_____

c) _____

_____

_____

_____

d) _____

_____

_____

_____

e) _____

_____

_____

_____

f) _____

_____

_____

_____

g) Turn on the water and adjust volume and temperature of water spray. Test the water temperature on inner wrist; monitor by keeping fingers under spray. Saturate the hair with warm water. Lift hair and work it with your free hand; protect the client's face, ears, and neck from the spray.

h) _____

_____

_____

_____

i) _____

_____

_____

_____

j) _____

_____

_____

_____

k) _____

_____

_____

_____

l) _____

_____

_____

_____

m) _____

_____

_____

_____

n) Allow the client's head to relax and work around the hairline with your thumbs in a rotary movement.

o) _____

_____

_____

_____

p) _____

_____

_____

_____

q) _____ 39

_____

_____

_____

r) _____

_____

_____

_____

s) _____

_____

_____

_____

t) _____

_____

_____

_____

u) _____

_____

_____

_____

v) Gently comb conditioner through, distributing it with a wide-tooth comb.

w) _____

_____

_____

_____

x) _____

_____

_____

_____

y) _____

_____

_____

_____

z) _____

_____

_____

_____

aa) Lift the towel and drape over the client's head by placing your hands on top of the towel and massaging until hair is partially dry. Ask the client to sit up.

bb) _____

_____

_____

_____

cc) _____

_____

_____

_____

dd) _____

_____

_____

_____

ee) Now you are ready to proceed with the rest of the service.

31. Why is it important to maintain good posture while performing a shampoo?

_____

_____

_____

32. What measures should you take to maintain good posture while shampooing, and why?

_____

_____

_____

33. What type of shampoo bowl allows for healthier body alignment and helps reduce back and shoulder strain?

_____

_____

34. List the typical types of hair.

a) _____

b) _____

c) _____

d) _____

35. Chemically treated hair may require products that are _____
_____ than products for hair that has not been chemically treated.

36. The amount of _____ in a solution determines whether that solution is alkaline or acidic.

37. A shampoo that is acidic will have a pH ranging from _____ to _____.

38. The more alkaline a shampoo, the stronger and harsher it is.

_____ True   _____ False

Rationale:

39. _____ is the most abundant and important element on Earth.

40. Why is water classified as a universal solvent?

_____

_____

41. Boiling water at a temperature of _____ degrees Fahrenheit will destroy most microbes.

42. _____ water is rainwater or chemically treated water that contains only small amounts of minerals, while _____ water contains minerals that reduce the ability of soap or shampoo to lather.

43. Generally, the main ingredient in most shampoos is _____ water, which has had impurities, such as calcium and magnesium and other metal ions, removed.

44. _____, also known as base detergents, are cleansing or surface active agents.

45. The end of a molecule that attracts water is called _____, while the oil-attracting end is called _____.

46. Shampoo products are the most widely purchased of all hair care products.

_____ True   _____ False

Rationale:

47. Many shampoos are pH balanced by adding _____, _____, or _____ acid.

48. _____ shampoos are designed to improve the manageability of the hair and make it appear smooth and shiny.

49. Give two examples of conditioning agents that boost shampoos.

1) _____

2) _____

50. Clarifying shampoos contain an active _____ agent that binds to metals and removes them from hair, as well as _____ agent that enriches hair, helps retain moisture, and makes hair more manageable.

51. Explain when clarifying shampoos should be used.

_____

_____

52. For oily hair and scalp, _____ shampoos wash away excess oiliness while preventing the hair from drying out.

53. A(n) _____ or _____ shampoo cleanses hair without soap and water.

54. A dry shampoo removes volume from hair.

_____ True   _____ False

Rationale:

55. Discuss the ways in which color-enhancing shampoos are used.

_____

_____

_____

56. Describe shampooing for wheelchair-bound clients.

_____

_____

_____

_____

_____

57. What implements and materials are required for a basic shampoo?

a) _____

b) _____

c) _____

d) _____

e) _____

f) _____

g) _____

h) _____

58. **ACTIVITY:** Gather a small group of at least five or six classmates to participate in this activity. Using Procedures 15–6 (Basic Shampooing and Conditioning) and 15–7 (Scalp Massage), write an abbreviated version of the procedural step on a piece of cardstock paper or construction paper. Do not number the steps. One procedure at a time, place all of the steps randomly around the floor of the classroom. Have each student attempt to place them in the proper order. The student who puts them in the proper order in the fastest amount of time gets the highest grade.

_____

_____

_____

_____

Recommend and Use Conditioners

59. Why are conditioners used?

_____

_____

60. Name the four basic types of conditioner.

1) _____

2) _____

3) _____

4) _____

61. Most conditioners contain silicone along with moisture-binding _____, substances that absorb moisture or promote the retention of moisture.

62. The cortex makes up _____ percent of the hair strand.

63. Identify some conditioning agents and their uses.

a) _____

_____

_____

b) _____

_____

_____

c) _____

_____

_____

d) _____

_____

_____

64. _____, also known as hair masks or conditioning packs, are chemical mixtures of concentrated protein and intensive moisturizer.

Use Professional Draping

65. Client draping contributes to the client's safety as well as comfort.

_____ True   _____ False

Rationale:

66. Name the two types of draping used in salons.

1) _____

2) _____

67. Explain when and how a shampoo draping is used.

_____

_____

_____

_____

_____

_____

_____

_____

68. When is a chemical draping used?

_____

_____

69. List the steps to draping for a chemical service.

a) _____

_____

_____

b) _____

_____

_____

c) _____

_____

_____

d) _____

_____

_____

e) _____

_____

_____

Understand the Benefits of the Three-Part Procedure

70. The pre-service procedure is an organized, step-by-step plan for which three tasks?

1) _____

2) _____

3) _____

71. List the three major tasks of the post-service procedure.

1) _____

2) _____

3) _____

CHAPTER 16 HAIRCUTTING

Date: _____

Rating: _____

Text Pages: 356–441

why study HAIRCUTTING?

1. In your own words, explain why cosmetologists should study and thoroughly understand haircutting.

   _____

   _____

   _____

   _____

   _____

   _____

   _____

   _____

   _____

Understand the Basic Principles of Haircutting

2. Good haircuts begin with an understanding of the _____, referred to as the _____.

3. To help achieve the look that you and your client are seeking, be aware of where the head form _____.

4. _____ on the head mark where the surface of the head changes.

5. List common reference points.

   a) _____   c) _____

   b) _____   d) _____

6. An understanding of head shape and reference points will help the cosmetologist in the following ways:

a) _____

_____

b) _____

_____

c) _____

_____

7. Match each of the following reference points with its description.

_____ Parietal ridge   a) Highest point on the top of the head

_____ Occipital bone   b) Widest area of the head, starting at the temples and ending at the bottom of the crown

_____ Apex   c) Front and back corners of the head

_____ Four corners   d) Bone that protrudes at the base of the skull

8. How can you find the parietal ridge? _____

_____

9. Describe how to find the occipital bone. _____

_____

10. Explain how to find the apex. _____

_____

11. Outline two ways to find the four corners. _____

_____

_____

_____

12. Name the areas of the head.

a) _____

b) _____

c) _____

d) _____

e) _____

f) _____

g) _____

13. Why is locating the parietal ridge important? _____

_____

_____

14. Give the procedure for determining the front of the head.

_____

_____

_____

15. Where are the sides of the head? _____

_____

16. What is the crown, and why is it important to identify? _____

_____

_____

_____

17. What is the nape, and how can it be identified? _____

_____

_____

_____

18. What does the back of the head consist of? Explain how to locate it.

_____

_____

19. Define the bang or fringe area. _____

_____

20. A(n) _____ is a thin, continuous mark used as a guide.

21. A(n) _____ is created when the space between two lines or surfaces intersects at a given point.

22. The two basic lines used in haircutting are:

1) _____

2) _____

23. Angles are important elements in creating a(n) _____

_____ in haircutting because this is how shapes are created.

24. Label the three types of straight lines in the accompanying figure:

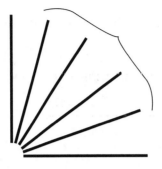

25. Horizontal lines are _____ ·from the floor and relative to the horizon.
    They _____ weight and are used to create _____ and
    _____ haircuts.

26. Vertical lines are _____ to the horizon. They _____
    weight to create _____ or layered haircuts and are used with
    _____ elevations.

27. Diagonal lines have a _____ direction and are used to create

_____.

28. _____ techniques use diagonal lines to create angles by cutting the
    ends of the hair with a slight increase or decrease in length.

29. For control during haircutting, the hair is parted into working areas called
    _____. Each section may be divided into smaller areas called

_____.

30. The line dividing the hair at the scalp, separating one section of hair from another, is
    called a _____ or _____.

31. List the four types of sections used in haircutting.

    1) _____

    2) _____

    3) _____

    4) _____

32. _____ is the degree at which a subsection of hair is held, or elevated,
    from the head when cutting.

33. In a blunt cut or one-length haircut, what degree of elevation is employed?

    _____ a) 90   b) 45   _____ c) 30   _____ d) 0

34. What are the two most commonly used elevations in haircutting?

1) _____

2) _____

35. The more you elevate the hair, the more _____ you create.

36. When you elevate hair below 90 degrees, you _____ weight.

37. When you elevate hair at 90 degrees or higher, you _____ weight.

38. _____ is when hair contracts or lifts through the action of moisture loss/drying.

39. The _____ is the angle at which the fingers are held when cutting the line that creates the end shape.

40. List the other names for the term cutting line.

a) _____

b) _____

c) _____

d) _____

41. Cutting lines can be described as:

a) _____

b) _____

c) _____

d) _____

42. Define the term guideline. _____

_____

43. The _____ of a cut is the outer line, while the _____ is the inner or internal line of the cut.

44. What are the two types of guidelines in haircutting?

1) _____

2) _____

45. A guideline that does not move during haircutting is considered _____.

46. A guideline that moves as a haircut progresses is classified as _____.

47. What is overdirection, and why is it used? _____

_____

_____

_____

_____

_____

Conduct an Effective Client Consultation for Haircutting

48. A _____ is a conversation between the cosmetologist and client during which the cosmetologist finds out what the client is looking for, offers suggestions and professional advice, and comes to a joint decision with the client about the most suitable haircut.

49. Explain how to analyze face shape. _____

_____

_____

_____

50. What does analyzing face shape accomplish? _____

_____

_____

_____

51. When analyzing face shape, an important point to consider is the client's _____, or how the client looks from the side.

52. What four characteristics determine the behavior of hair?

1) _____

2) _____

3) _____

4) _____

53. The _____ is the hair that grows at the outermost perimeter along the face, around the ears, and on the neck.

54. The growth pattern is the direction in which the hair grows from the scalp, also called the _____ or the _____.

55. You may need to use _____ tension when cutting cowlicks, whorls, and other growth patterns to compensate for hair being pushed up when it dries.

_____ a) more   _____ b) less

56. The number of individual hair strands on 1 square inch (2.5 cm²) of scalp is known as

_____.

57. _____ is usually classified as coarse, medium, or fine and is based on the thickness or diameter of each strand.

58. Why are density and texture important? _____

_____

_____

59. The _____, or the amount of movement in a hair strand, can be completely straight, wavy, curly, extremely curly, or anything in between.

Show Proper Use of Haircutting Tools

60. Match each of the following tools with its most common haircutting use.

_____ Haircutting shears   a) To achieve a softer effect on the ends of the hair

_____ Texturizing shears   b) To remove excess or unwanted neckline hair

_____ Razors   c) For close tapers when using the scissor-over-comb technique

_____ Clippers   d) To detangle hair

_____ Trimmers   e) To cut blunt or straight lines

_____ Sectioning clips   f) To section and subsection hair

_____ Wide-tooth comb   g) For most haircutting procedures

_____ Tail comb   h) Come in a variety of shapes, styles, and sizes

_____ Barber comb   i) Create short haircuts, tapers, fades, and flat tops

_____ Styling or cutting comb   j) To remove bulk from the hair

61. 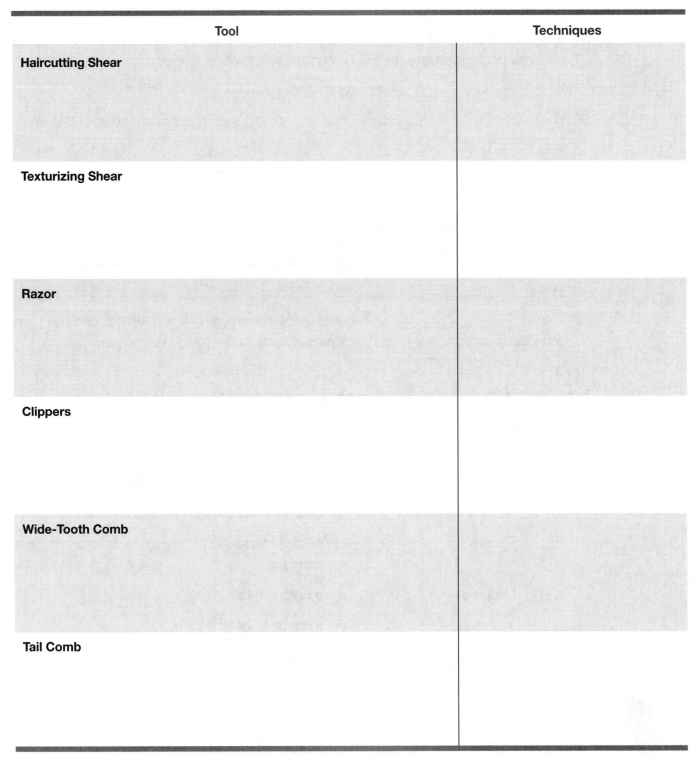 **ACTIVITY:** Complete the following chart by drawing a picture of each of the tools listed, labeling each key part, and describing techniques that can be accomplished with each tool.

Tool	Techniques
Haircutting Shear	
Texturizing Shear	
Razor	
Clippers	
Wide-Tooth Comb	
Tail Comb	

62. Which three countries are primarily responsible for manufacturing the steel used to make professional shears?

1) _____ 2) _____ 3) _____

63. Generally, a shear with a Rockwell hardness of at least _____ or _____ is ideal.

64. As the strength or hardness of the steel increases, the shear's ability to retain a sharp edge:

    _____ a) increases.   _____ b) decreases.   _____ c) remains the same.

65. A(n) _____ shear is made by pouring molten steel into a mold, whereas a(n) _____ shear is made by a process of working metal into a finished shape by hammering or pressing.

66. Compare forged shears with cast ones. _____

    _____

    _____

    _____

    _____

67. Match each of the following shear parts with its function.

    _____ Cutting edge   a) Affords more shear control

    _____ Pivot and adjustment area   b) Does the cutting

    _____ Adjustment knob   c) Make the shears cut

    _____ Finger tang   d) Pulls the blades together at the correct tension

68. List all the tasks that should be on the shears' maintenance schedule.

    a) _____

    b) _____

    c) _____

    d) _____

    e) _____

69. A left-hand cutter can use a right-handed shear by simply turning the shear over.

    _____ True   _____ False

    ┌───┐
    │ Rationale: │
    │   │
    │   │
    │   │
    │   │
    └───┘

70. Name the things a cosmetologist should look for when considering a shears purchase.

a) _____

b) _____

c) _____

d) _____

e) _____

f) _____

g) _____

h) _____

i) _____

j) _____

k) _____

71. When purchasing shears, a full _____ edge will give the smoothest cut, while a(n) _____ edge is dull and can be noisy.

72. Which of the following types of shears adds increased blending?

_____ a) Chunking   _____ c) Thinning

_____ b) Texturizing   _____ d) Blending

73. Ergonomically correct and custom-fitted shears can help the cosmetologist dramatically by:

a) _____

b) _____

c) _____

74. List the four components of correctly fitting a shear.

1) _____

2) _____

3) _____

4) _____

75. It is important to hold tools properly because doing so:

a) _____

b) _____

76. Describe the important elements of holding shears.

a) _____

_____

b) _____

_____

c) _____

_____

77. Why is it important to always hold the comb while cutting?

_____

_____

_____

78. Differentiate between the roles of the dominant hand and the holding hand during

haircutting. _____

_____

_____

_____

79. Explain what it means to "palm the shears." _____

_____

_____

_____

80. Define the phrase *transferring the comb*. _____

_____

_____

_____

81. A(n) _____, or feather blade, is a versatile tool that can be used for an
entire haircut.

82. Describe the two methods of holding a razor.

Method A

a) _____

_____

b) _____

_____

c) _____

_____

Method B

a) _____

b) _____

83. In a comb, _____ teeth are used for combing and parting hair, while _____ teeth comb a section before cutting.

84. In haircutting, _____ is the amount of pressure applied when combing and holding a subsection.

85. Why is consistent tension important in haircutting? _____

_____

Understand Proper Posture and Body Position

86. What steps can you take to ensure you are using good posture and body positioning when cutting hair?

a) _____

b) _____

c) _____

87. List the hand positions for different cutting angles and when they are used.

a) _____

_____

b) _____

_____

c) _____

_____

88. Describe the cutting technique and line being used in the image below.

_____

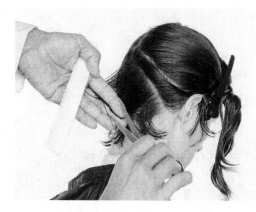

Maintain Safety in Haircutting

89. What precautions should you take when handling sharp tools and instruments?

a) _____

_____

b) _____

_____

c) _____

_____

d) _____

_____

e) _____

_____

Cut Hair Using Basic Haircutting Techniques

90. Name the four basic haircuts.

1) _____

2) _____

3) _____

4) _____

91. In a(n) _____ cut, also known as a one-length haircut, all the hair comes to a single hanging level, forming a weight line.

92. What is a weight line? _____

_____

93. Which of the following apply to a cutting line in a blunt cut? Mark all that apply.

_____ a) Horizontal   _____ b) Diagonal   _____ c) Rounded

94. The most common elevation in a graduated haircut is _____ degrees.

_____ a) 180   _____ b) 90   _____ c) 45   _____ d) 0

95. A(n) _____ haircut is an effect achieved by cutting the hair with elevation or overdirection.

96. A layered haircut is cut at higher elevations, usually _____ degrees.

_____ a) 180   _____ b) 90   _____ c) 45   _____ d) 0

97. A long-layered haircut is ultimately cut at a _____ -degree elevation.

_____ a) 180   _____ b) 90   _____ c) 45   _____ d) 0

98. Describe the shape of a long-layered haircut. _____

_____

99. List general haircutting tips. The first answer is provided to get you started.

a) Always make consistent and clean partings.

b) _____

_____

c) _____

_____

d) _____

_____

e) _____

_____

f) _____

_____

g) _____

_____

h) _____

_____

i) _____

_____

j) _____

_____

k) _____

_____

l) _____

_____

k) _____

_____

100. _____ is parting the haircut in the opposite way that you cut it, at the same elevation, to check for precision of line and shape.

101. Give some alternate names for the blunt cut. _____

_____

102. For a blunt cut, the client's head should be in what position?

_____

_____

_____

103. What happens when a client's head is improperly positioned with the head forward for a blunt cut?

a) _____

b) _____

104. Identify the implements, materials, and supplies needed for the blunt cut.

a) _____

b) _____

c) _____

d) _____

e) _____

f) _____

g) _____

h) _____

i) _____

j) _____

k) _____

l) _____

m) _____

105. How should the hair be parted when cutting a blunt cut? _____

_____

_____

106. Where do you begin a blunt haircut? _____

_____

_____

107. When cutting the sides behind the ear in a blunt cut, what should you pay close

attention to? _____

_____

108. In a blunt cut, how do you check the line for accuracy? _____

_____

_____

109. In a classic A-line bob, a(n) _____ forward cutting line is
used.

110. In a classic pageboy, the perimeter is _____, using a combination of
horizontal and curved diagonal back lines.

111. List tips for blunt haircuts.

a) _____

b) _____

c) _____

d) _____

e) _____

f) _____

112. In the basic _____ haircut, you will be utilizing vertical, horizontal, and diagonal cutting lines with a 45-degree elevation at the back and 90-degree elevation for the layers.

113. Describe the type of haircut depicted in the following illustration and the techniques used to create it. _____

_____

_____

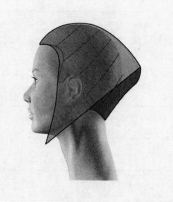

114. In a uniform-layered haircut, all hair is elevated to _____ degrees from the scalp and cut at the same length, using a(n) _____ guideline that is inside the haircut rather than on the perimeter.

115. List the steps involved in completing a long-layered haircut *right handed*. Some steps have been filled in to help you out.

a) _____

b) _____

c) _____

_____

_____

d) Detangle the hair with the wide-tooth comb.

e) _____

_____

_____

_____

f) _____

_____

_____

g) Take another ½-inch (1.25 cm) wide set of slight diagonal forward subsections from the top of the occipital to the top of each ear. The head position will move up slightly, but the natural fall distribution and 0-degree elevation will remain. Cut parallel to the parting and following the length of your guide.

h) _____

_____

_____

i) _____

_____

_____

j) _____

_____

_____

k) _____

_____

l) _____

_____

_____

m) To keep the length on the sides from front to back, avoid cutting your corner at the sideburn area or just in front of the ear. Clients with long hair want to see their length at the front and back.

n) _____

_____

_____

o) _____

_____

_____

p) _____

_____

_____

q) _____

_____

r) Once the sides are completed and you've checked your balance, take two diagonal forward partings at the top of the occipital to the back of each ear. The hair below your diagonal parting will be sectioned out of the way.

s) _____

_____

t) _____

_____

_____

u) _____

_____

_____

_____

v) _____

_____

_____

w) _____

_____

x) _____

_____

_____

y) Section the hair the same manner it was cut and blowdry using a large round brush.

z) Once the hair is dry, detail the interior and perimeter using deep point cutting. Hold the section 3 inches (7.5 centimeters) from the ends and enter the hair parallel (use the entire length of the blade) so you don't remove any length.

aa) _____

_____

Understand Other Cutting Techniques

116. What is important to remember when cutting curly hair? _____

_____

_____

117. Curly hair can appear shorter after it dries because of a _____ effect. For every ¼ inch (0.6 centimeters) you cut when the hair is wet, it will shrink up to _____ inch when dry.

118. Why should you use minimal tension when cutting curly hair?

_____

_____

119. What is the effect of using a razor on curly hair?

_____

_____

120. The _____ or _____ area includes the hair that lies between the two front corners, or approximately between the outer corners of the eyes.

121. What is meant by distribution? _____

_____

122. A razor cut gives a _____ appearance than a shear cut.

123. Differentiate between a shear cut and a razor cut. _____

_____

_____

124. A razor guide is _____ your fingers, whereas the guide with shears is usually _____ your fingers.

125. Why should you always use a new, sharp blade when razor cutting?

_____

_____

126. List tips for cutting with a razor.

a) _____

b) _____

c) _____

d) _____

e) _____

127. Slide cutting is useful for:

a) _____

b) _____

c) _____

128. How is slide cutting accomplished? _____

_____

129. _____ is a technique in which you hold the hair in place with a comb while using the tips of shears to remove length.

130. The scissor-over-comb technique is generally used to:

a) _____

b) _____

131. List the basic steps of the shears-over-comb technique.

a) _____

_____

b) _____

_____

c) _____

_____

_____

d) _____

_____

132. What comb is used to cut areas very close such as sideburns and hairlines where the hair is cut close to the scalp?

_____

133. _____ is the process of removing excess bulk without shortening the length.

134. Texturizing techniques can be used to:

a) _____

b) _____

c) _____

d) _____

135. What tools are used for texturizing? _____

_____

136. Match each of the following texturizing techniques with the phrase that best describes it.

_____ Point cutting	a) More aggressive method of point cutting creating a chunkier effect
_____ Notching	b) Thins hair to graduated lengths with shears
_____ Free-hand notching	c) Removes weight and adds movement through lengths of hair
_____ Effilating	d) Creates a broken edge
_____ Slicing	e) Creates a visual separation in the hair
_____ Carving	f) Used on the interior of the section to release curl and remove density

137. When discussing texturizing, what might be a better choice of words than thinning?

_____

138. What is the razor rotation technique used for? _____

_____

139. Describe the action taking place in the following image of a razor haircut:

_____

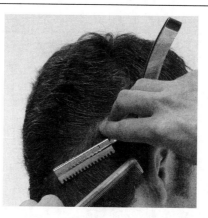

Effectively Use Clippers and Trimmers

140. What are clippers? _____

_____

141. Clippers are good for cutting shorter haircuts and can be used to create a
_____, hair that is cut very short and close to the hairline and gradually
gets longer as you move up the head.

142. Identify the ways in which clippers can be used.

a) _____

_____

b) _____

_____

c) _____

_____

143. List all the tools to have on hand when clipper cutting.

a) _____

b) _____

c) _____

d) _____

e) _____

144. Describe the action taking place in the following photo.

_____

_____

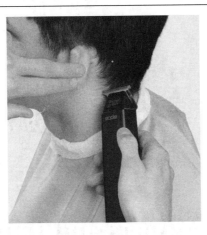

145. The _____ technique allows you to cut very close to the scalp and create a flat top or square shape.

146. Clippers are more accurate when used on _____ hair.

147. Always work against the natural growth pattern when cutting with clippers.

_____ True   _____ False

Rationale:

148. When using the clipper-over-comb technique, the angle at which you hold the comb determines the _____.

149. Using the length guard attachments is a quick and easy way to create _____ haircuts.

150. Clippers and trimmers can be used to trim beards and mustaches.

_____ True   _____ False

Rationale:

151. How should you part the hair for a men's basic clipper cut?

_____

_____

_____

_____

152. Where and how should you begin the men's basic clipper cut?

_____

_____

_____

_____

153. In a men's basic clipper cut, how do you eliminate any corners in your design line?

_____

_____

_____

_____

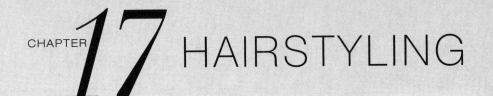

CHAPTER 17 | HAIRSTYLING

Date: _____

Rating: _____

Text Pages: 442–525

why study HAIRSTYLING?

1. In your own words, explain why cosmetologists should study and thoroughly understand hairstyling.

_____

_____

_____

_____

_____

_____

_____

_____

_____

Start with a Client Consultation

2. What is the best way for clients to convey their expectations in terms of hairstyle preference?

_____

_____

3. What factors will help determine the best hairstyle?

_____

_____

_____

Learn the Basics of Wet Hairstyling

4. List the commonly used wet hairstyling tools.

a) _____

b) _____

c) _____

d) _____

e) _____

f) _____

Perform Finger Waving

5. Finger waving is the process of _____
through the use of the fingers, combs, and finger-waving lotion.

6. Why should cosmetologists learn finger waving of the 1920s and 1930s?

_____

_____

_____

_____

7. _____ is a type of hair gel that makes the hair pliable enough to keep it
in place during the finger-waving procedure.

8. Finger-waving lotion is traditionally made from _____, taken from trees
found in _____ and _____.

9. How will you know if you have used too much finger-waving lotion on the hair?

_____

10. How do vertical finger waves differ from horizontal finger waves?

_____

_____

11. List the implements and materials needed for wet hairstyling.

a) _____

b) _____

c) _____

d) _____

e) _____

12. Describe the action in the image below.

_____

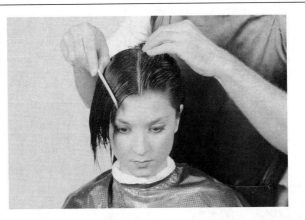

13. Describe how to create a part.

a) _____

b) _____

c) _____

14. List the implements and materials needed for horizontal finger waving.

a) _____

b) _____

c) _____

d) _____

e) _____

f) _____

g) _____

h) _____

i) _____

j) _____

k) _____

15. How should you apply waving lotion during horizontal finger waving?

_____

_____

16. Horizontal finger waving should begin where?

_____ a) Forehead   c) Nape

_____ b) Hairline   d) Ear

17. To begin the formation of the first ridge during horizontal finger waving, place the index finger of your non-dominant hand directly above the position for the first ridge. With the teeth of the comb pointing _____, insert the comb directly under the index finger.

18. In horizontal finger waving, the first and second ridges are created using the same movements.

_____ True   _____ False

Rationale:

19. What does the accompanying figure illustrate?

_____

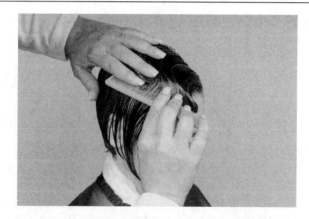

20. Once an entire head is finger waved, what should you do?

_____

_____

_____

21. How do you achieve a retro look upon finishing horizontal finger waving?

_____

_____

_____

Form Pin Curls

22. _____ serve as the basis for patterns, lines, waves, and rolls that are used in a wide range of hairstyles.

23. Pin curls can be used only on hair that has been permanently waved.

_____ True   _____ False

Rationale:

24. Pin curls work best when the hair is layered and smoothly wound.

_____ True   _____ False

Rationale:

25. Identify the three principal parts of pin curls shown in the image below.

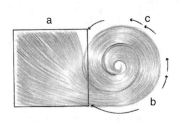

a) _____

b) _____

c) _____

26. The _____ is the stationary _____ foundation of the curl, which is the area closest to the scalp.

27. The _____ is the section of the pin curl between the base and first arc _____ of the circle that gives the curl its direction and movement.

28. The size of the _____, determines the width of the wave and its strength.

29. The _____ is the hair between the scalp and the first turn of the roller.

_____ a) base   _____ b) stem   _____ c) circle

30. The amount of mobility, or movement, in a section of hair is known as the

_____.

31. The _____ curl is placed directly on the base of the curl. It produces a tight, firm, long-lasting curl and allows minimum mobility.

32. The _____ curl permits medium movement; the curl is placed half off the base and gives good control to the hair.

33. The _____ curl allows for the greatest mobility because the curl is placed completely off the base and gives as much freedom as the length of the stem will permit.

34. The base of a full-stem curl may be of what shape?

_____

_____

35. A(n) _____ is a section of hair that is molded in a circular movement in preparation for the formation of curls.

36. Shapings are either _____ or _____.

37. _____ curls produce even, smooth waves and uniform curls.

38. _____ curls produce waves that get smaller toward the ends.

39. What is a clockwise curl?

_____

_____

40. What is a counterclockwise curl?

_____

_____

41. What base shapes are used in pin curls?

a) _____

b) _____

c) _____

d) _____

42. To avoid splits in a finished hairstyle, use care when selecting and forming the

_____.

43. Where are rectangular base pin curls recommended?

_____

_____

44. Where are triangular base pin curls recommended?

_____

_____

45. How are arc base pin curls made, and where are they used?

_____

_____

46. When are square base pin curls used?

_____

_____

47. To avoid splits when combing out a square base pin curl set, you should _____ the sectioning.

48. _____ is the technique that involves forcing the hair between the thumb and the back of the comb to create tension.

_____ a) Threading   c) Slicing

_____ b) Ribboning   d) Sculpting

49. Pin curls sliced from a shaping and formed without lifting the hair from the head are called _____ curls, also known as _____ curls.

50. How are pin curls used to create ridge curls?

_____

_____

51. What are skip waves?

_____

_____

52. _____ curls have large center openings and are fastened to the head in a standing position on a rectangular base.

53. What effect do barrel curls give?

_____

_____

54. What are cascade curls used for?

_____

_____

55. How are cascade curls fastened?

_____

_____

56. What implements and materials are needed for a wet set with rollers?

a) _____

b) _____

c) _____

d) _____

e) _____

f) _____

g) _____

h) _____

i) _____

j) _____

k) _____

l) _____

57. To begin the wet set, you should _____

_____.

58. For a wet set, start at the _____ and part off a section the same length and width as the roller.

59. In a wet set with rollers, what factor determines what type of base to use?

_____

_____

60. How is the hair held when wrapping it around a roller?

_____

_____

Create Roller Curls

61. What advantages do rollers have over pin curls?

a) _____

_____

b) _____

_____

c) _____

_____

62. Identify the three parts of the roller curl.

1) _____

2) _____

3) _____

62. What is the function of the base in a roller curl?

_____

64. What is the appropriate size of a roller curl base?

_____

65. In a roller curl, the _____ is the hair between the scalp and the first turn of the roller.

66. What is the function of the stem in a roller curl?

_____

67. In a roller curl, the _____, or circle, is the hair that is wrapped around the roller.

68. Why is the size of a roller curl circle important?

_____

69. Match the following type of curl with the number of times it is wound around the roller.

_____ One complete turn   a) Curls

_____ One and a half turns   b) C-shaped curl

_____ Two and a half turns   c) Wave

70. The amount of _____ that is achieved depends on the size of the roller and how the roller sits on its base.

71. An on-base curl will give _____ volume.

72. A half-base curl will give _____ volume.

73. A(n) _____ curl will give the least volume.

74. For versatility in styling, a(n) _____ directional wrap gives options to style in all directions while still maintaining volume.

75. _____ is the point where curls of opposite directions meet, forming a recessed area.

76. Hot rollers are to be used only on dry hair.

_____ True   _____ False

Rationale:

77. What type of client is best suited for a Velcro™ set?

_____

_____

78. Why do the state boards of some states and provinces disallow Velcro rollers?

_____

_____

79. How long do Velcro rollers stay in the hair?

_____

_____

80. 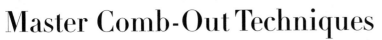 **ACTIVITY:** Section your mannequin hair into four sections by making a part from the center front hairline to the center of the nape and then from the top of one ear over the apex to the top of the other ear. In the front left section of the mannequin, use on-base rollers and no-stem pin curls to set the hair. In the front right section, use half-base rollers and half-stem pin curls to set the hair. In the back left section, use off-base rollers and full-stem pin curls to set the hair. In the back right section, use any combination of pin curls and roller placements you desire. Dry the mannequin completely. Then, attempt to complete a comb out and analyze the differences in each section based on the types of curls used. Consider how the different curls impact the finished look.

_____

_____

_____

_____

_____

_____

_____

Master Comb-Out Techniques

81. What are the benefits of a well-structured system of combing out hairstyles?

_____

_____

82. What techniques are used to lift and increase volume, give direction, as well as remove the indentations caused by roller setting?

_____

_____

83. List the alternative names for backcombing.

a) _____

b) _____

c) _____

d) _____

84. What action is involved in backcombing?

_____

_____

85. _____, or ruffing, is used to build a soft cushion or to mesh two or more curl patterns for a uniform and smooth comb out.

86. For what purposes are backcombing and backbrushing used today?

_____

_____

87. List the steps for the backcombing technique.

a) _____

b) _____

c) _____

d) _____

e) _____

f) _____

88. List the steps for the backbrushing technique.

a) _____

b) _____

c) _____

d) _____

e) _____

f) _____

89. When is a finishing spray applied during backbrushing?

_____

_____

Understand Hair Wrapping

90. What is the purpose of hair wrapping?

_____

_____

91. When height is desired with hair wrapping, place large rollers _____,
with the remainder of the hair wrapped around the head.

92. Wrapping can be done on wet hair only.

_____ True   _____ False

Rationale:

93. When wrapping very curly hair, the first step is to _____.

94. List the implements and materials needed for hair wrapping.

a) _____

b) _____

c) _____

d) _____

e) _____

f) _____

g) _____

h) _____

i) _____

j) _____

95. What product is applied to dry hair before wrapping?

_____

96. To begin hair wrapping, where is the first parting created?

_____

97. During hair wrapping, starting on the heavy side of the part, using a
_____ paddle brush, begin to wrap hair smooth to head shape
_____or in desired style direction.

98. While wrapping, use _____ or large bobby pins to keep the hair in place.

99. When all the hair is wrapped, _____

_____ .

100. When working on dry hair, leave the hair wrapped for about _____ minutes.

101. When wrapping wet hair, place the client under a hooded dryer until the hair is completely dry, usually _____ minutes to one hour, depending on the _____ .

Finish Hair Using Basic Blowdry Styling

102. Blowdry styling is the technique of _____ and _____ damp hair in one operation.

103. A(n) _____ is an electrical appliance designed for drying and styling hair.

104. The blowdryer's nozzle attachment, or _____ , is a directional feature that creates a concentrated stream of air.

105. The _____ of a blowdryer is an attachment that causes the air to flow more softly and helps to accentuate or keep textural definition.

106. What can happen when a blowdryer is not clean?

_____

107. Combs and picks are designed to _____ and _____ the hair.

108. Combs with teeth that are closely spaced _____ definition from the curl and create a smooth surface.

109. Combs with widely spaced teeth _____ larger sections of hair for a more textured surface.

110. Combs with a pick at one end _____ .

111. Describe a classic styling brush.

_____

_____

112. What are classic styling brushes best used for?

_____

_____

_____

113. Describe a paddle brush and what it is used for.

_____

_____

_____

114. _____ brushes are generally oval with a mixture of boar and nylon bristles.

115. In a grooming brush, _____ bristles help distribute the scalp oils over the hair shaft, giving it shine, while _____ bristles stimulate the circulation of blood to the scalp.

116. What are grooming brushes particularly useful for?

_____

_____

_____

117. _____ brushes, with their ventilated design, are used to speed up the blowdrying process and are ideal for blowdrying fine hair and adding lift at the scalp.

118. How are the various sizes of round brushes used?

_____

_____

_____

119. Why do some round brushes have metal cylinder bases?

_____

_____

_____

120. A(n) _____ brush is a nylon styling brush that has a tail for sectioning, along with a narrow row of bristles.

121. How are teasing brushes used?

_____

_____

_____

122. _____ clips are usually metal or plastic and have long prongs to hold wet or dry sections of hair in place.

123. Styling products can be thought of as _____ tools.

124. What options must stylists consider before applying styling products?

a) _____

b) _____

c) _____

d) _____

125. Foam builds _____ body and volume into the hair.

126. How is mousse used?

_____

_____

127. Foam is good for which type of hair? Why?

_____

128. What is the purpose of gel?

_____

_____

129. How do liquid gels relate to firm hold gels?

_____

_____

130. Explain the effect of straightening gels.

_____

_____

131. When sprayed into the roots of fine, wet hair that is then blown dry, _____ add volume, especially at the base.

132. _____, also known as wax, adds considerable weight to the hair by causing strands to join together, showing separation in the hair.

133. Non-oily silicone products are excellent for all hair types, either to provide lubrication and protection to the hair during blowdrying, or to finish a style by adding extra shine.

_____ True   _____ False

Rationale:

134. Hair spray, also known as _____ spray, is applied in the form of a mist to hold a style in position.

135. Products that protect the hair from heat damage caused by thermal styling tools like blowdryers, flat irons, and curling irons are called _____

_____.

136. List the implements and materials needed for blowdrying short, layered, or curly hair to produce a smooth and full finish.

a) _____

b) _____

c) _____

d) _____

e) _____

f) _____

g) _____

h) _____

i) _____

j) _____

k) _____

137. List the steps to blowdry short, layered, curly hair to produce a smooth and full finish once a clean neck strip is in place. The first step has been filled in to help you get started.

a) Remove any tangles with a wide-tooth comb, starting at the ends and working up to the scalp.

b) _____

_____

c) _____

_____

d) _____

_____

e) _____

_____

f) _____

_____

_____

g) _____

_____

_____

h) _____

_____

_____ .

i) _____

_____

_____ .

138. What does the accompanying figure illustrate?

_____

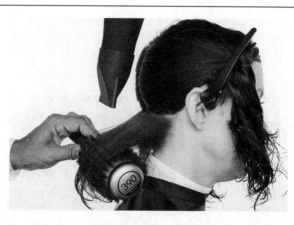

139. List the steps to diffuse long, curly, or extremely curly hair in its natural wave pattern once a clean neck strip is in place. The first step has been filled in to help you get started.

a) Remove any tangles with a wide-tooth comb, starting at the ends and working up to the scalp.

b) _____

_____

_____

_____

c) _____

_____

_____

_____

d) _____

_____

_____

_____

e) _____

_____

_____

_____

f) _____

_____

_____

_____

140. List the steps to blowdry blunt or long-layered, straight to wavy hair into a straight style once a light gel or a straightening gel is applied. The first step has been filled in to help you get started.

a) Attach the nozzle or concentrator attachment to the blowdryer for more controlled styling. Part and section the hair so that only the section you are drying is not in clips.

b) _____

_____

_____

_____

c) _____

_____

_____

_____

d) _____

_____

_____

_____

e) _____

_____

_____

_____

f) _____

_____

_____

_____

g) _____

_____

_____

_____

h) _____

_____

_____

_____

i) _____

_____

_____

_____

j) _____

_____

_____

_____

141. What does the accompanying figure illustrate? _____

_____

Maintain Safety in Thermal Hairstyling

142. Thermal waving and curling is also called _____ waving.

143. Explain what is meant by thermal waving and curling?

_____

_____

_____

144. Which stylists favor nonelectrical thermal irons, and why?

_____

_____

_____

145. Name the four basic parts of a thermal iron.

1) _____   3) _____

2) _____   4) _____

146. Flat irons with straight edges are used to create _____ styles, even on very curly hair.

147. What is the best way to test an iron's temperature?

_____

_____

_____

148. Describe how to remove dirt, oils, or product residue from a thermal iron.

_____

_____

_____

_____

149. The comb used with a thermal iron should be about _____ inches long.

_____ 3 (7.5 centimeters)   _____ 7 (17.5 centimeters)

_____ 5 (12.5 centimeters)   _____ 9 (22.5 centimeters)

150. Describe how to hold a thermal iron.

a) _____

_____

b) _____

_____

c) _____

_____

151. What factor determines the correct temperature for thermal styling?

_____

_____

152. As a rule, coarse and gray hair can withstand _____ heat than fine hair.

153. Why is thermal curling used on straight hair?

_____

_____

154. Thermal curling cannot be used on human hair wigs and hairpieces.

_____ True   _____ False

Rationale:

155. What is the key to becoming good at using curling irons?

_____

_____

156. Developing a smooth _____ movement is important in thermal curling.

157. When practicing with thermal irons, guiding the hair strand into the center of the curl as you rotate the irons helps ensure that _____

_____.

158. How can you protect the client's scalp from burns while removing a curl from a thermal iron?

_____

159. The _____ curl is a method of curling the hair by winding a strand around the rod.

160. The spiral curl creates a _____ effect and works best on one length hair to create volume.

161. The _____ creates volume of hair, movement, and a curl formation from roots to ends that is commonly used on short or long layered hair.

162. What are end curls? _____

_____

163. What factors determine whether end curls turn under or over?

_____

_____

164. _____ thermal iron curls stem from the root curl and are used to create volume or lift in a finished hairstyle.

165. What determines the type of volume curls to be used?

_____

_____

166. Match each of the following base curl types with the volume it provides.

_____ Volume-base   a) Moderate

_____ Full-base   b) Slight

_____ Half-base   c) Maximum

_____ Off-base   d) Full

167. Why do volume-base curls provide maximum lift or volume?

_____

_____

168. How is a volume-base curl wound?

_____

_____

_____

_____

_____

169. Explain how to wind full-base curls.

_____

_____

_____

_____

_____

170. What result can you expect to get with a half-base curl?

_____

171. Outline the procedure for winding a half-base curl.

_____

_____

_____

_____

_____

172. A(n) _____ curl is placed completely off its base and offers a curl option with only slight lift or volume.

173. When a hairstyle is to be finished with curls, brush the _____ curls last.

174. _____ combs must not be used in thermal curling as they are flammable.

175. Allowing hair ends to protrude over a thermal iron causes _____, hair that is bent or folded.

176. List the implements and materials needed for thermal waving.

a) _____

b) _____

c) _____

d) _____

e) _____

f) _____

g) _____

177. In thermal waving, what factor determines whether the first wave is left-moving or right-moving?

_____

_____

178. During thermal waving, how much hair should be picked up before inserting the iron?

_____

_____

179. Where should the groove of the iron be when you insert it into the hair?

_____

180. Once the iron is in the hair, what should you do? _____

_____

_____

181. What does the accompanying figure illustrate?

_____

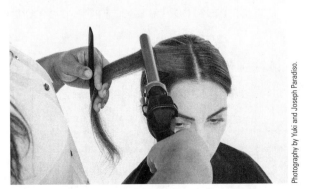

Photography by Yuki and Joseph Paradiso.

Thermal Hair Straightening (Hair Pressing)

182. When done properly, _____ temporarily straightens extremely curly or resistant hair by means of a heated iron or comb.

183. How long does a pressing last?

_____

184. What additional services can hair pressing prepare the hair for?

_____

_____

185. A good hair pressing leaves the hair in a _____ condition.

186. Match each of the following pressing types with the percentage of curl it removes from hair.

_____ Soft   a) 60 to 75

_____ Medium   b) 100

_____ Hard   c) 50 to 60

187. A _____ press is accomplished by applying the thermal pressing comb once on each side of the hair.

188. A hard press, which involves applying a thermal pressing comb _____ on each side of the hair, is also called a _____ press.

189. Before pressing a client's hair, analyze the condition of the _____ and

_____ .

190. When a client's hair and scalp are unhealthy, what should you do?

_____

_____

191. Failure to correct _____ hair can cause hair breakage during hair pressing.

192. What two things must you check before agreeing to give a pressing?

_____

_____

193. A careful analysis of a client's hair should cover what points?

a) _____

b) _____

c) _____

d) _____

e) _____

f) _____

g) _____

h) _____

194. Why is it important for the cosmetologist to be able to recognize individual differences in hair texture, porosity, elasticity, and scalp flexibility?

_____

_____

_____

_____

195. Variations in hair texture have to do with the _____ of the hair and the _____ of the hair.

196. Which hair texture has qualities that make it difficult to press?

_____

197. Coarse, extremely curly hair requires less heat and pressure than medium or fine hair in the pressing process.

_____ True _____ False

Rationale:

198. Medium curly hair is the most resistant to hair pressing.

_____ True _____ False

Rationale:

199. To avoid breaking fine hair, use less heat and pressure than for other hair textures.

_____ True   _____ False

Rationale:

200. What does wiry, curly hair feel like?

_____

201. What makes wiry hair resist hair pressing?

_____

_____

202. Wiry hair requires _____ heat and pressure than other types of hair.

203. List the three possible conditions of a client's scalp.

1) _____

2) _____

3) _____

204. If the scalp is tight and the hair coarse, how should you press the hair?

_____

205. What should the cosmetologist remember with a flexible scalp?

_____

_____

206. During the client consultation, the cosmetologist should ask the client about which of the following elements? Check all that apply.

_____ a) Lightener   _____ d) Gradual colors metallic

_____ b) Client's age   _____ e) Other chemical treatments

_____ c) Tint

207. As with all services, the client should sign a _____ before hair pressing in order to protect the school, the salon, and the stylist from liability due to accidents or damage.

208. Effective _____ involve special cosmetic preparations for the hair and scalp, thorough brushing, and scalp massage.

209. Explain how to make a tight scalp more flexible.

_____

_____

210. What are the two types of pressing combs?

_____

211. What should pressing combs be made of?

_____

212. A pressing comb with closely spaced teeth provides a _____ press.

213. Pressing combs are all the same size.

_____ True   _____ False

```
Rationale:



```

214. Why should you temper a new pressing comb made of brass?

_____

_____

215. How should you temper a new pressing comb?

_____

_____

_____

216. When heating a pressing comb in a gas stove, point the teeth _____ and keep the handle _____ from the fire.

217. How will you know when a pressing comb is too hot?

_____

_____

218. Electric pressing combs are available in what two forms?

a) _____

b) _____

219. Describe how to clean a pressing comb.

_____

_____

220. How can you remove carbon from a pressing comb?

_____

_____

_____

_____

221. List the benefits of pressing oil or cream.

a) _____

b) _____

c) _____

d) _____

e) _____

f) _____

g) _____

222. When is a hard press recommended?

_____

_____

223. A hard press is also known as a(n) _____ press.

224. What may cause pressed hair to curl again?

_____

_____

225. The cosmetologist can prevent the smoking or burning of hair during a pressing treatment by _____

_____.

226. In the event of an accidental burn during pressing, what should the cosmetologist do immediately?

_____

_____

227. When pressing coarse hair, apply enough pressure so that the hair remains

_____.

228. When pressing lightened or tinted hair, the client may need _____

_____.

229. Because gray hair may resist pressing, use a _____ pressing comb applied with _____ pressure.

Creatively Style Long Hair

230. Describe an updo.

_____

_____

231. Name three classic updo techniques.

1) _____

2) _____

3) _____

232. Identify the five key points that must be considered before you begin an updo, also known as a specialty style.

1) _____

2) _____

3) _____

4) _____

5) _____

233. The two basic hairstyles that are the foundation of every updo and long hairstyling are the _____.

234. List the implements and materials needed to style a chignon.

a) _____

b) _____

c) _____

d) _____

e) _____

f) _____

g) _____

h) _____

i) _____

j) _____

k) _____

l) _____

k) _____

l) _____

235. How should you secure the ponytail of a knot or chignon?

_____

_____

236. Explain how to conceal the elastic band of a knot or chignon.

_____

_____

_____

237. When creating a chignon, how should you secure the left and right undersides of the roll? _____

238. List the steps to create a french pleat or twist after the hair has been blown dry. The first step has been filled in to help you get started.

a) Set the hair with a wet set or, if you wish to save time, electric rollers or thermal irons.

b) _____

_____

_____

_____

_____

c) _____

_____

_____

_____

d) _____

_____

_____

_____

e) _____

_____

_____

_____

f) _____

_____

_____

_____

g) _____

_____

_____

_____

h) _____

_____

_____

_____

i) _____

_____

_____

_____

_____

j) _____

_____

_____

_____

k) _____

_____

_____

_____

_____

239. Describe what is depicted in the image below.

_____

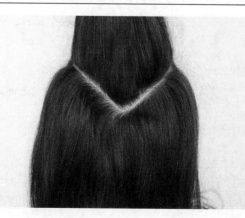

Perform Formal Styling

240. When performing a pre-wedding consultation, always suggest _____ styles for the bride and leave the latest trend for the bridesmaids.

Date: _____

Rating: _____

Text Pages: 526–569

Know the General History of Braiding

1. Historically, the first highly decorative braids were seen among _____ tribes.

2. Today, braids are as acceptable as any other hairstyle in most modern workplaces.

   _____ True   _____ False

Rationale:

3. Braiding salons practice what is commonly known as _____ hairstyling, which uses no chemicals or dyes and does not alter the natural curl or coil pattern of the hair.

4. With proper care, a braided hair design can last up to _____ months, with _____ to _____ weeks being preferable.

5. What is the best way to avoid miscommunications and misunderstandings and ensure a happy ending to every natural styling service?

   _____

why study BRAIDING AND BRAID EXTENSIONS?

6. In your own words, explain why cosmetologists should study and have a thorough understanding of the importance of braiding and braid extensions.

_____

_____

_____

_____

_____

_____

_____

_____

_____

Understand the Basics of Braiding

7. When analyzing the condition of a client's hair and scalp during consultation, you should pay particular attention to the hair's _____, curl configuration, scalp abrasions, and hair thinning or balding.

8. In braiding and other natural hairstyling, texture refers to what three qualities?

   1) _____

   2) _____

   3) _____

9. In addition to texture, the cosmetologist should consider what characteristics during hair analysis?

   a) _____

   b) _____

   c) _____

   d) _____

   e) _____

   f) _____

   g) _____

   h) _____

10. Everyone has thinner, finer hair around the hairline.

_____ True _____ False

Rationale:

11. In the natural hairstyling and braiding world, hair is referred to as _____ or _____ if it has never had any chemical treatments.

12. _____ involves overlapping two strands of hair to achieve a candy cane effect.

13. Sewing a weft of faux or natural hair onto a cornrow braid is known as _____.

14. Some states have separate natural hairstyling licenses.

_____ True _____ False

Rationale:

15. Stylists who hold only braiding, natural hairstyling, or locktician licenses can perform such chemical services as coloring or relaxing.

_____ True _____ False

Rationale:

16. Identify the tools used for braiding. The first tool has been filled in to help you get started.

a) Boar-bristle brush or natural hairbrush.

b) _____

c) _____

d) _____

e) _____

f) _____

g) _____

h) _____

i) _____

j) _____

k) _____

l) _____

m) _____

n) _____

o) _____

p) _____

q) _____

r) _____

17. What is the advantage of using a boar-bristle brush?

_____

_____

_____

18. Explain the use of the square paddle brush in braiding.

_____

_____

_____

_____

19. In braiding, the vent brush is used to _____

_____ .

20. The distance between teeth is the most important feature of a wide-tooth comb.

_____ True   _____ False

Rationale:

21. Which of the following tools is excellent for design parting, sectioning large segments of hair, and opening and removing braids?

_____ a) Diffuser   _____ c) Tail comb

_____ b) Long clip   _____ d) Finishing comb

22. Identify the implements and materials needed for extensions:

a) _____

b) _____

c) _____

23. What is a hackle? _____

_____

_____

24. _____ are flat leather pads with very close, fine teeth that sandwich human hair extensions.

25. The fibers used for the purpose of extending hair largely determine how successful and durable the extension will be.

_____ True   _____ False

Rationale:

26. List some materials commonly used for hair extensions.

a) _____

b) _____

c) _____

d) _____

e) _____

f) _____

27. What is Kanekalon, and why is it a good choice for extensions?

_____

_____

_____

_____

28. Discuss the pros and cons of nylon or rayon synthetic.

_____

_____

_____

_____

_____

29. Why is traditional yarn now being used to adorn hair?

_____

_____

_____

_____

_____

30. Why should care be taken when purchasing yarn?

_____

_____

_____

_____

_____

31. _____, a beautiful wool fiber imported from Africa, has a matte finish and comes only in black and brown.

32. The strong fiber that comes from the domestic ox found in the mountains of Tibet and Central Asia is _____.

33. Why is it best to braid curly hair when it is dry?

_____

_____

_____

_____

34. Straight, resistant hair is best braided slightly damp or very lightly coated with _____ or _____ to make it more pliable.

35. Textured hair is very fragile both wet and dry.

_____ True   _____ False

Rationale:

36. List all of the implements, materials, and supplies needed to prepare textured hair for braiding. The first item has been filled in to help you get started.

a) Blowdry cream or lotion with botanical, essential oils.

b) _____

c) _____

d) _____

e) _____

f) _____

g) _____

h) _____

i) _____

j) _____

37. When preparing textured hair for braiding, part the back of the head into _____ to _____ sections. For thick, textured hair, make _____ sections; for thinner hair, use _____ sections.

38. Explain how to blowdry the client's hair as part of the procedure for preparing textured hair for braiding.

_____

_____

_____

_____

_____

Braid the Hair

39. _____ braids are three-stand braids created with a(n) _____ technique in which the left section goes under the middle strand, then the right section goes under the middle strand.

40. _____ or _____ braids are three-strand braids produced with a(n) _____ technique in which the first side section goes over the middle one, then the other side section goes over the middle strand.

41. What type of braid is created with two strands that are twisted around each other?

_____

42. The _____ braid is a simple, two-strand braid in which hair is picked up from the sides and added to the strands as they are crossed over each other.

43. The fishtail braid is best done on layered hair that is at least shoulder length.

_____ True   _____ False

Rationale:

44. What does the accompanying figure illustrate? _____

_____

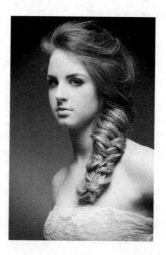

45. The _____ are two or three long, simple inverted thick cornrows created around the head.

46. The invisible braid is ideal for long hair, but it can be executed on shorter hair with long layers.

_____ True _____ False

Rationale:

47. What do the terms single braids, box braids, and individual braids refer to?

_____

_____

_____

48. The partings or subsections for single braids can be what shape?

a) _____ c) _____

b) _____ d) _____

49. With single braids, the _____ determines where the braid is placed and how it moves.

50. Extensions for single braids come in a wide range of sizes and lengths and are integrated into the natural hair using the _____ technique.

51. Fibers for extensions can be selected from _____, _____, or _____.

52. Discuss the client consultation and the process for preparing a client for a single braid with extensions.

_____

_____

_____

_____

_____

_____

53. What are the steps in the procedure for creating single braids with extensions? Some steps have been filled in to help you out.

a) _____

_____

b) _____

_____

c) _____

_____

d) Apply a light essential oil to the scalp, and massage it into the scalp and throughout the hair.

e) _____

_____

f) _____

_____

_____

_____

_____

g) _____

_____

h) _____

_____

_____

i) Divide the natural hair into three equal sections. Place the folded extension on top of the natural hair, on the outside and center portions of the braid.

j) _____

_____

_____

_____

_____

k) _____

_____

l) _____

_____

m) _____

_____

_____

n) _____

_____

_____

_____

_____

o) _____

_____

_____

p) After the entire head has been braided, remove all loose hair ends from the braid shaft with shears.

q) _____

_____

_____

54. _____, also called _____, are narrow rows of visible braids that lie close to the scalp.

55. How are cornrows created? _____

_____

56. How long do cornrows last? _____

_____

57. Explain why the feed-in method is used for cornrows with extensions.

_____

_____

_____

_____

_____

58. Compare traditional cornrows with those created with the feed-in method.

_____

_____

_____

_____

_____

_____

59. Give some options for finishing basic cornrows.

_____

_____

_____

_____

_____

60. Outline the procedure for creating basic cornrows. Some steps have been filled in to help you out.

a) Drape the client for a shampoo. If necessary, comb and detangle the hair before shampooing.

b) _____

_____

_____

_____

c) _____

_____

_____

_____

d) _____

_____

_____

e) _____

_____

_____

_____

f) _____

_____

_____

g) _____

_____

_____

h) _____

_____

_____

i) _____

_____

_____

j) _____

_____

_____

_____

k) _____

_____

_____

l) Repeat until all the hair is braided and apply oil sheen for shine.

61. Explain the technique of tree braiding and how tree braids are created.

_____

_____

_____

_____

_____

_____

62. ⓦ **ACTIVITY:** Conduct an Internet search for "natural braiding hairstyles" and look through the many, many styles found. Magazines are another source for these pictures. Select at least six styles and mount the braided looks onto a poster board. Under each style, describe the type of braid used and any particular techniques or procedures you believe were required to create the look. Then select at least two of the looks and attempt to duplicate the look on your mannequin or a willing model.

_____

_____

_____

Classify Textured Sets and Styles

63. List and explain the techniques for textured sets and styles below.

a) _____

_____

_____

_____

b) _____

_____

_____

_____

c) _____

_____

_____

d) _____

_____

_____

_____

e) _____

_____

_____

_____

f) _____

_____

_____

_____

64. What are locks? _____

_____

_____

65. List and briefly explain the four basic methods of locking.

1) _____

_____

_____

2) _____

_____

_____

3) _____

_____

_____

4) _____

_____

_____

Date: _____

Rating: _____

Text Pages: 570–595

1. The _____ shaved their heads with bronze razors and wore heavy black wigs to protect themselves from the sun.

2. In ancient _____, women wore wigs made from the prized blond hair of barbarians captured from the North.

3. In eighteenth-century England, men wore wigs, called _____, to indicate that they were in the army or navy, or engaged in the practice of law.

4. Most clients today have their wigs custom fitted.

    _____ True   _____ False

Rationale:

5. Toupees are often custom-made and fitted.

    _____ True   _____ False

Rationale:

why study WIGS AND HAIR ADDITIONS?

6. In your own words, explain why cosmetologists should study and thoroughly understand wigs and hair additions. _____

_____

_____

_____

_____

_____

_____

_____

Establish the Differences Between Human and Synthetic Hair

7. Describe the fastest way to tell if a hair strand is synthetic or human.

_____

_____

_____

_____

8. List the advantages of human hair.

a) _____

b) _____

c) _____

9. List the disadvantages of human hair.

a) _____

   _____

b) _____

   _____

c) _____

   _____

d) _____

   _____

10. List the advantages of synthetic hair.

a) _____

b) _____

c) _____

d) _____

e) _____

f) _____

g) _____

h) _____

11. List the disadvantages of synthetic hair.

a) _____

b) _____

c) _____

d) _____

12. The more expensive wigs, hairpieces, and extensions are those made of human hair.

_____ True   _____ False

Rationale:

13. European hair is at the top of the line.

_____ True   _____ False

Rationale:

14. Color-treated hair is more costly than virgin hair.

_____ True   _____ False

Rationale:

15. What two regions of the world provide most of the human hair commercially available?

_____ a) India and South America   _____ c) Asia and North America

_____ b) Middle East and India   _____ d) India and Asia

16. Indian hair is usually available in lengths from _____ to _____ inches.

_____ a) 3 to 7   _____ c) 12 to 16

_____ b) 8 to 12   _____ d) 12 to 28

17. Asian hair is available in lengths from _____ to _____ inches.

_____ a) 3 to 7   _____ c) 12 to 16

_____ b) 8 to 12   _____ d) 12 to 28

18. Indian hair is naturally _____, whereas Asian hair is naturally

_____.

19. What types of animal hair are mixed with human hair to create wigs?

_____

20. Mixed-hair products are often used in which of the following?

_____ a) Hair competitions   _____ c) Theatrical settings

_____ b) Cancer patients   _____ d) Bridal updos

21. What questions should you ask when selecting a hair addition for a client?

a) _____

_____

b) _____

_____

c) _____

_____

d) _____

_____

e) _____

_____

f) _____

_____

g) _____

_____

h) _____

_____

i) _____

_____

j) _____

_____

22. What is turned hair? _____

_____

_____

23. Define the term fallen hair. _____

_____

_____

_____

Learn Basic Wig Knowledge

24. A _____ can be defined as an artificial covering for the head consisting of a network of interwoven hair.

25. If a hair addition does not fully cover the head, it is either a(n) _____, which is a small wig used to cover the top or crown of the head, or a hair _____ of some sort.

26. Name the two basic categories of wigs.

1) _____

2) _____

27. _____ wigs are constructed with an elasticized, mesh-fiber base to which the hair is attached.

28. How are cap wigs sized? _____

_____

29. What does it mean if a cap wig is hand-knotted? _____

_____

30. How are cap wigs constructed and made to fit the head? _____

_____

_____

_____

31. _____ wigs are machine-made from human or artificial hair.

32. Long strips of hair with a threaded edge are known as _____.

33. Why are capless wigs more popular than cap wigs? _____

_____

34. Capless wigs are extremely light and comfortable to wear due to their
    _____ and _____.

35. What type of client is a cap wig best suited for, and why?

_____

_____

36. Match each of the following wigs with its description.

_____ Hand-tied or hand-knotted wig	a) Made by feeding wefts through a sewing machine and then stitching them together to form the base and shape of the wig
_____ Semi-hand-tied wig	b) Made by inserting individual strands of hair into a mesh foundation and knotting them with a needle
_____ Machine-made wig	c) Constructed with a combination of synthetic hair and hand-tied human hair

37. Explain why is it important to be aware of the artificial growth patterns of a wig.

_____

_____

38. The most flexible and versatile of all patterns is the _____ wig.

39. _____ wigs are sewn in a specific direction, offering no versatility.

40. The creation of a custom-made wig begins with _____

_____.

41. Most wig manufacturers ask for precise specifications of what characteristics?

a) _____

b) _____

c) _____

d) _____

42. Why do ready-to-wear wigs require no measuring? _____

_____

_____

43. Many wigs need to be adjusted to the head and _____ to suit the client.

44. When measuring the head for a wig, make sure to _____

_____ in order to lay the tape measure gently around the head.

45. A _____ is a head-shaped form, usually made of canvas-covered cork or Styrofoam, on which the wig is secured for fitting, coloring, and sometimes styling.

46. The block is best attached to the work area with a swivel clamp, which allows for greater control.

_____ True   _____ False

Rationale:

47. Today, most wigs are cut and finished while on the block.

_____ True   _____ False

Rationale:

48. Describe the proper procedure for putting on a wig. _____

_____

_____

_____

49. When cutting a wig, generally the goal is to _____

_____.

50. When cutting and trimming wigs, what basic methods of haircutting can you follow?

_____

_____

_____

51. When free-form cutting, vertical sections create _____, diagonal
    sections create a(n) _____ edge, and horizontal sections build
    _____.

52. Free-form cutting is usually done on dry hair, which allows you to see how the hair will
    fall.

    _____ True   _____ False

Rationale:

53. Compare the wet cutting method with the dry cutting method.

_____

_____

54. Often, the more abstract cutting method results in a cut that looks less realistic.

    _____ True   _____ False

Rationale:

55. When using heat on a human hair wig, always set the styling tool to what position?

_____ Low _____ Medium _____ High

56. Traditionally, brushes made with _____ have been regarded as best for use on human hair.

57. Comb-outs and finishing touches for most modern cuts should be done on the block.

_____ True _____ False

Rationale:

58. For a wig to look believable, what three areas must appear the most convincing?

1) _____

2) _____

3) _____

59. To style a wig to look as natural as possible, always follow the direction of the

_____.

60. What type of styling products should be used for the hairline?

_____

61. To make the hairline of a wig look natural, you should _____ gently around the hairline.

62. What is a wind test? _____

_____

_____

63. When styling a wig, you should make the final results look perfect.

_____ True _____ False

Rationale:

64. What is the best way to clean any wig? _____

_____

_____

_____

_____

_____

65. What is the most common color level of wigs? Why?

_____

_____

66. If you are going to custom color wig hair, use hair that has been decolorized through the
_____ process, not with _____ dyes.

67. The first step when coloring a wig is to _____.

68. Hair in which the cuticle is absent is very _____ and will react to color in
an extreme manner.

69. Always _____ the hair prior to a full-color application.

70. When coloring a wig, what color products can be used?

a) _____

b) _____

c) _____

d) _____

e) _____

71. When coloring a human hair wig or hair addition, conduct regular color checks every
_____ to _____ minutes.

72. Often, it is easier to color a client's hair to match a hair addition than to color the
addition itself.

_____ True   _____ False

Rationale:

73. You may safely perm wig hair that has been colored with a metallic dye.

_____ True   _____ False

Rationale:

74. Where should an addition be while performing a permanent wave?

_____

_____

_____

Know the Different Types of Hairpieces

75. What is a hairpiece, and how much coverage does it give?

_____

_____

76. List some different types of hairpieces.

a) _____

b) _____

c) _____

77. A(n) _____ hairpiece has openings in the base, through which the client's own hair is pulled to blend with the _____ hair of the hairpiece.

78. Integration hairpieces are very lightweight, natural-looking products that add _____ and _____ to the client's hair.

79. A(n) _____ is a small wig used to cover the top and crown of the head.

80. What are the two ways to attach toupees?

1) _____

2) _____

81. _____ hairpieces, which include ponytails, chignons, cascades, streaks, bangs, falls/half wigs, and clip-in hair extensions, are a great salon product for special occasions or for use as fashion accessories.

82. Fashion hairpieces vary in _____ and are constructed on a

_____.

83. Identify five temporary means for attaching fashion hairpieces.

1) _____

2) _____

3) _____

4) _____

5) _____

84. ACTIVITY: Take a field trip to a local wig shop or salon. Visit with the proprietor or salesperson to see the various types and styles of wigs. Learn which wigs are the most popular sales items and find out why. Complete the form below about at least six different wigs or hairpieces.

Type of Wig or Hairpiece	Construction	Color	Material Used	Style	Care Required	Cost

_____

_____

Study the World of Hair Extensions

85. _____ are hair additions that are secured to the base of the client's natural hair to add length, volume, texture, or color.

86. What general guidelines should you keep in mind when attaching hair extensions?

a) _____

_____

b) _____

_____

c) _____

_____

d) _____

_____

e) _____

_____

f) _____

_____

87. Name some ways to attach hair additions.

a) _____

b) _____

c) _____

d) _____

e) _____

88. The most important professional approaches to hair addition and extension services should be practiced in the following order:

a) _____

b) _____

c) _____

d) _____

89. In the _____, hair extensions are secured to the client's own hair by sewing braids or a weft onto an on-the-scalp braid or cornrow, which is sometimes called the _____.

90. In the braid-and-sew method, the _____ of the track determines how the hair will fall.

91. Identify the directions in which tracks may be positioned in the braid-and-sew method.

a) _____

b) _____

c) _____

d) _____

92. In the braid-and-sew method, it is best to place the tracks or braids _____ inch(es) behind the hairline to ensure proper coverage.

93. How are extensions sewn onto a track in the braid-and-sew method?

_____

_____

_____

_____

94. Name the stitches that may be used to sew extensions to a track.

a) _____

c) _____

b) _____

95. _____ involves attaching hair extensions, hair wefts or single strands with an adhesive or bonding agent.

96. Generally, bonding product will last from _____ to _____ weeks.

97. What factors affect how long hair will remain bonded?

a) _____

b) _____

c) _____

98. Discuss the advantages of bonding. _____

_____

_____

_____

_____

99. What do the accompanying figures depict? _____

_____

_____

_____

_____

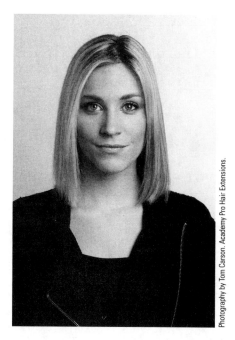

Photography by Tom Carson. Academy Pro Hair Extensions.

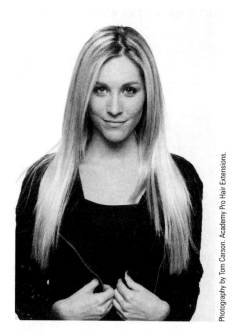

Photography by Tom Carson. Academy Pro Hair Extensions.

100. In the _____ method of attaching extensions, individual extension hair is bonded to the client's own hair with a bonding material that is activated by the heat from a special tool.

101. What are the advantages of the fusion-bonding method?

a) _____

_____

b) _____

_____

c) _____

_____

102. How long do fused attachments last?_____

_____

103. Some fusion-bonding procedures involve wrapping a(n) _____ strip around both the client's hair and the extension.

104. Explain the disadvantages of fusion bonding. _____

_____

_____

_____

105. Give an overview of the linking process. _____

_____

_____

_____

106. Usually the problems with tube shrinking arise from the materials, not the stylist or client.

_____ True   _____ False

Rationale:

107. What are some guidelines for retailing hair goods or offering hair-addition services?

a) _____

_____

b) _____

_____

c) _____

_____

d) _____

_____

e) _____

_____

f) _____

_____

g) _____

_____

20 CHEMICAL TEXTURE SERVICES

Date: _____

Rating: _____

Text Pages: 596–667

why study CHEMICAL TEXTURE SERVICES?

1. In your own words, explain why cosmetologists should study and thoroughly understand chemical texture services. _____

   _____

   _____

   _____

   _____

   _____

   _____

   _____

   _____

   _____

   _____

2. _____ are hair services that cause chemical changes within the hair's natural wave and curl pattern.

3. Identify some chemical texture services.

   a) _____

   b) _____

   c) _____

Understand How Chemical Services Affect the Structure of Hair

4. Name the three layers of the hair.

   1) _____

   2) _____

   3) _____

5. The cuticle is directly involved in the texture or movement of the hair.

   _____ True   _____ False

Rationale:

6. The medulla does not play a role in chemical texture services and may be missing in fine hair.

   _____ True   _____ False

Rationale:

7. The natural pH of hair is between _____ and _____.

8. Chemical solutions _____ the pH of the hair to an alkaline state.

9. Coarse, resistant hair with a strong, compact cuticle layer requires a highly alkaline chemical solution.

   _____ True   _____ False

Rationale:

10. List the basic building blocks of hair.

a) _____

b) _____

c) _____

d) _____

e) _____

11. _____ bonds, also known as end bonds, are chemical bonds that join amino acids together, end-to-end in long chains, to form a polypeptide chain.

12. Side bonds are _____, _____, and _____ bonds that cross-link polypeptide chains together.

13. Disulfide bonds can be broken by boiling water.

_____ True   _____ False

Rationale:

14. Disulfide bonds are the weakest of the three side bonds.

_____ True   _____ False

Rationale:

15. Salt bonds are broken by changes in pH.

_____ True   _____ False

Rationale:

16. Individual hydrogen bonds are very weak.

_____ True   _____ False

Rationale:

17. Water easily breaks _____ bonds, and these bonds re-form as the hair dries or cools.

Demonstrate the Proper Technique for Permanent Waving

18. _____ is a two-step process whereby the hair undergoes a physical change caused by wrapping the hair on perm rods, and then undergoes a chemical change by applying permanent waving solution and neutralizer.

19. You should always perform an elasticity test before perming the hair.

_____ True   _____ False

Rationale:

20. In permanent waving, what two factors determine curl size?

1) _____

2) _____

21. Alkaline permanent waving solutions soften and swell the hair.

_____ True   _____ False

Rationale:

22. Name the four reactions that occur in the chemical process of permanent waving.

1) _____

_____

_____

2) _____

_____

_____

3) _____

_____

_____

4) _____

_____

_____

23. All permanent wave solutions contain a reducing agent.

_____ True   _____ False

Rationale:

24. _____, a colorless liquid with a strong, unpleasant odor, is the most common reducing agent in permanent wave solutions.

25. The alkalinity of the perm solution should correspond to the _____, _____, and _____ of the cuticle layer.

26. Alkaline waves have a pH between _____ and _____.

27. _____ is the main active ingredient in true acid and acid-balanced waving lotions.

28. List the three components of all acid waves.

1) _____

2) _____

3) _____

29. Explain how a true acid wave, with a pH below 7.0, can cause the hair to swell.

_____

_____

_____

_____

30. Pure water can damage the hair.

_____ True _____ False

Rationale:

31. Discuss the effect of higher pH on acid-balanced waves.

_____

_____

_____

32. An exothermic chemical reaction absorbs heat.

_____ True _____ False

Rationale:

33. Give two examples of alkanolamines that are used in permanent waving solutions as substitutes for ammonia.

1) _____

2) _____

34. Permanents based on sulfites are very weak and do not provide firm curls, especially on strong or resistant hair.

_____ True   _____ False

Rationale:

35. Hair that has been treated with a semipermanent color is not as porous as hair treated with permanent color and may actually appear more resistant.

_____ True   _____ False

Rationale:

36. Which of the following perm types is recommended for extremely porous hair?

_____ a) Alkaline/cold wave   _____ c) True acid wave

_____ b) Thio-free wave   _____ d) Exothermic wave

37. Explain how the strength and processing amount of a permanent wave process is

determined. _____

_____

_____

38. _____ is essential to ensure proper processing for all permanent waves.

39. A properly processed permanent wave should break and rebuild approximately _____ percent of the hair's disulfide bonds.

40. Overprocessed hair is overly curly.

_____ True   _____ False

Rationale:

41. Underprocessed hair is usually straighter at the scalp and curlier at the ends.

_____ True   _____ False

Rationale:

42. In permanent waving, _____ stops the action of the waving solution and rebuilds the hair into its new curly form.

43. Identify the two functions of neutralization.

1) _____

2) _____

44. The most common neutralizer is _____.

45. Give some tips for proper rinsing and blotting during thio neutralization.

a) _____

_____

b) _____

_____

c) _____

_____

d) _____

_____

e) _____

_____

f) _____

_____

g) _____

_____

h) _____

_____

i) _____

_____

j) _____

_____

46. Identify the information preliminary test curls provide.

a) _____

b) _____

c) _____

d) _____

e) _____

f) _____

g) _____

47. Name the implements, materials, and supplies needed to perform a preliminary test curl for a permanent wave. A few items are listed to help you get started.

a) Applicator bottles.

b) Chemical cape.

c) _____

d) _____

e) _____

f) _____

g) _____

h) _____

i) _____

j) _____

k) _____

l) _____

m) _____

n) Pre-neutralizing conditioner (optional).

o) _____

p) _____

q) _____

r) _____

s) _____

t) _____

48. _____ rods produce a tighter curl in the center and a looser curl on either side of the strand.

49. Soft bender rods are usually about _____ long with a uniform diameter along the entire length of the rod.

50. End papers should extend beyond the ends of the hair to prevent _____, hair that is bent up at the ends.

51. Name the most common end-paper techniques.

a) _____

b) _____

c) _____

52. What is the purpose of the double flat wrap? _____

_____

_____

53. The _____ wrap eliminates excess paper and can be used with short rods or with very short lengths of hair.

54. _____ are subsections of panels into which the hair is divided for perm wrapping.

55. Explain how base placement is determined. _____

_____

56. Using a base section that is wider than the perm rod can create an uneven curl pattern and undue tension on the hair.

_____ True   _____ False

Rationale:

57. In which type of base placement is the hair wrapped at a 90-degree angle?

_____ a) On-base   _____ b) Half off-base   _____ c) Off-base

58. _____ refers to the angle at which the rod is positioned on the head.

59. A _____ wrap is wrapped from the ends to the scalp in overlapping concentric layers.

60. In a spiral perm wrap, the hair is wrapped perpendicular to the length of the rod.

_____ True   _____ False

Rationale:

61. List six perm wrapping patterns.

1) _____

2) _____

3) _____

4) _____

5) _____

6) _____

62. The _____ is the position of the tool in relation to its base section, determined by the angle at which the hair is wrapped.

63. In the procedure for permanent wave and processing using a basic permanent wrap, you divide the hair into _____ panels.

64. What is the proper procedure for wrapping panels in permanent wave and processing using a basic permanent wrap?

a) _____

_____

_____

b) _____

_____

_____

c) _____

_____

_____

65. Discuss the sectioning procedure for permanent wave and processing using a curvature permanent wrap. _____

_____

_____

_____

_____

66. Outline the procedure for permanent wave and processing using a bricklay permanent wrap. The first step is provided to help you get started.

a) After completing the pre-service procedure, seat the client. If the manufacturer's directions indicate a shampoo is necessary before the service, then drape the client for a shampoo and gently shampoo and toweldry hair. Avoid irritating the client's scalp.

b) _____

_____

_____

_____

c) _____

_____

_____

_____

d) _____

_____

_____

_____

e) _____

_____

f) _____

_____

_____

_____

g) _____

_____

_____

_____

h) _____

_____

_____

_____

i) _____

_____

_____

_____

j) _____

_____

_____

_____

67. The _____ technique uses zigzag partings to divide base areas.

68. What is the procedure for permanent wave and processing using a weave double-rod or piggyback technique? The first step is provided to help you get started.

a) After completing the pre-service procedure, seat the client. If the manufacturer's directions indicate a shampoo is necessary before the service, then drape the client for a shampoo and gently shampoo and towel-dry hair. Avoid irritating the client's scalp.

b) _____

_____

_____

c) _____

_____

_____

d) _____

_____

_____

e) _____

_____

_____

f) _____

_____

_____

g) _____

_____

_____

h) _____

_____

_____

i) _____

_____

_____

j) _____

_____

_____

k) _____

_____

_____

69. Name all the implements, materials, and supplies needed for a permanent wave and processing using a spiral wrap technique. The first and last items are listed to help you get started.

a) Applicator bottles.

b) _____

c) _____

d) _____

e) _____

f) _____

g) _____

h) _____

i) _____

j) _____

k) _____

l) _____

m) _____

n) _____

o) _____

p) _____

q) _____

r) _____

s) _____

t) Towels.

70. Partial perms can be used for what kinds of clients?

a) _____

_____

b) _____

_____

c) _____

_____

71. What additional considerations are there for partial perms?

a) _____

_____

_____

b) _____

_____

_____

72. Why are many male clients requesting perms?

a) _____

b) _____

c) _____

d) _____

73. What benefits can perming provide for male clients?

a) _____

b) _____

c) _____

74. The techniques for permanent waving men's hair differ from those used on women.

_____ True   _____ False

Rationale:

75. List the safety precautions for permanent waving. The first safety precaution is provided to help you get started.

a) Always protect your client's clothing. Have the client change into a gown, or use a waterproof chemical cape, and double drape with towels to absorb accidental spills.

b) _____

_____

c) _____

_____

d) _____

_____

e) _____

_____

f) _____

_____

g) _____

_____

h) _____

_____

i) _____

_____

j) _____

_____

k) _____

_____

l) _____

_____

m) _____

_____

n) _____

_____

76. Some home haircoloring products contain _____ that are not compatible with permanent waving because they leave a coating on the hair that may cause uneven curls, severe discoloration, or hair breakage.

Demonstrate the Proper Technique for Chemical Hair Relaxers

77. _____ is a process that rearranges the structure of curly hair into a straighter or smoother form.

78. What are the most common types of chemical hair relaxers?

   a) _____

   b) _____

   c) _____

79. In extremely curly hair, the thinnest and weakest sections are at the twists.

   _____ True   _____ False

Rationale:

80. _____ is the measurement of the thickness or thinness of a liquid that affects how the fluid flows.

81. The chemical reactions of thio relaxers differ from those used in permanent waving.

   _____ True   _____ False

Rationale:

82. Explain how to avoid scalp irritation when applying thio relaxer to virgin hair.

   _____

   _____

83. Discuss the proper procedure for applying thio relaxer to virgin hair once protective base cream has been applied. _____

   _____

   _____

   _____

_____

_____

_____

_____

_____

_____

84. For a thio relaxer retouch, divide the hair into _____ sections.

85. Explain what to do during a thio relaxer retouch once the relaxer has been applied to all sections. The first step is provided to help you get started.

a) Use the back of the comb, the applicator brush, or your hands to smooth each section.

b) _____

_____

_____

_____

_____

_____

c) _____

_____

_____

_____

_____

_____

d) _____

_____

_____

_____

_____

_____

e) _____

_____

_____

_____

_____

_____

f) _____

_____

_____

_____

_____

_____

g) _____

_____

_____

_____

_____

_____

h) _____

_____

_____

_____

_____

_____

i) _____

_____

_____

_____

86. What is the general procedure for Japanese thermal straighteners?

_____

_____

_____

_____

_____

_____

_____

87. Hydroxide relaxers are compatible with thio relaxers, permanent waving, and soft curl perms.

_____ True   _____ False

Rationale:

88. The average pH of the hair is _____, and many hydroxide relaxers have a pH _____.

89. In _____, the process by which hydroxide relaxers permanently straighten hair, the relaxers remove a sulfur atom from a disulfide bond and convert it into a lanthionine bond.

90. Identify the types of hydroxide relaxers.

a) _____

b) _____

c) _____

91. What are the two most common low-pH relaxers?

1) _____

2) _____

92. _____, also known as protective base cream, is an oily cream used to protect the skin and scalp during hair relaxing.

93. Protective base cream should always be applied to the entire scalp, hairline, and around the ears, even with no-base relaxers.

_____ True   _____ False

Rationale:

94. Most chemical relaxers are available in what three strengths?

1) _____

2) _____

3) _____

95. What is the purpose of periodic strand testing? _____

_____

96. Unlike thio neutralization, _____ is an acid-alkali neutralization that neutralizes (deactivates) the alkaline residues left in the hair by a hydroxide relaxer and lowers the pH of the hair and scalp.

97. Since the scalp area and the porous ends usually process more quickly than the middle of the strand, the application for a virgin relaxer starts _____ to _____ away from the scalp and includes the entire strand up to the porous ends.

98. What is the proper way to apply hydroxide relaxer to virgin hair after you have applied the protective base cream? _____

_____

_____

_____

_____

_____

_____

_____

_____

_____

99. Keratin alone will straighten hair.

_____ True   _____ False

```
Rationale:




```

100. How do keratin straightening treatments work?

_____

_____

101. Pre-conditioning before a keratin straightening treatment is meant to

_____

102. If a client wishes to have a demi-gloss treatment, it should be done at least
_____ to _____ days after the keratin treatment.

Demonstrate the Proper Technique For Curl Re-Forming (Soft Curl Permanents)

103. What is curl re-forming? _____

_____

104. A(n) _____ is a thio-based chemical service that reformats curly and wavy hair into looser and larger curls and waves.

105. By what other name is a soft curl permanent called?

_____

106. List the materials, implements, and supplies needed for curl re-forming (soft curl perm). The first item is listed to help you get started.

a) Applicator bottle.

b) _____

c) _____

d) _____

e) _____

f) _____

g) _____

h) _____

i) _____

j) _____

k) _____

l) _____

m) _____

107. Give some safety precautions for hair relaxing and curl re-forming. The first two safety precautions are listed to help you get started.

a) Perform a thorough hair analysis and client consultation prior to the service. Hair should be in relatively good condition.

b) Examine the scalp for abrasions. Do not proceed with the service if redness, swelling, or skin lesions are present.

c) _____

_____

d) _____

_____

e) _____

_____

f) _____

_____

g) _____

_____

h) _____

_____

i) _____

_____

j) _____

_____

k) _____

_____

l) _____

_____

m) _____

_____

n) _____

_____

o) _____

_____

p) _____

_____

q) _____

_____

r) _____

_____

s) _____

_____

t) _____

_____

108. The first step in the soft curl permanent procedure is to _____

_____.

109. During a soft curl perm, after the hair has been processed and the Thio cream has been rinsed thoroughly, towel blot the hair and part it into _____ panels.

110. Use the length of the _____ to measure the width of the panels.

111. Where should you begin wrapping? _____

_____

112. Wearing gloves, apply Thio wrap lotion to each _____ and roll hair on the appropriate-sized perm rods.

113. What size should the horizontal partings be? _____

_____

114. Hold the hair at a _____ angle to the head. Using two end papers, roll the hair down to the scalp and position the rod _____.

115. Place cotton strip around the _____ to protect the client.

116. When processing is completed, rinse the hair thoroughly for at least _____, and then gently towel blot each rod to _____.

117. Apply the _____ slowly and carefully to each rod.

118. ACTIVITY: After shampooing, conditioning, and detangling your mannequin, perform a four-section T-parting. Wrap each section with a different style and size rod. Also use different types of end wraps on each section for practice. Dry the mannequin thoroughly, remove the rods, and comb through each section with a wide-tooth comb. Compare the various curl patterns. Consider how these different curl patterns will affect the various styles you may perform in the salon. After you have completed your analysis, apply a mock application of relaxer on the curliest section and have your instructor grade your application technique.

_____

_____

_____

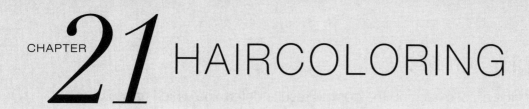

CHAPTER 21 HAIRCOLORING

Date: _____

Rating: _____

Text Pages: 668–733

1. Clients who have their hair colored usually visit the salon every _____ to _____ weeks.

why study HAIRCOLORING?

2. In your own words, explain why cosmetologists should study and thoroughly understand hair coloring.

_____

_____

_____

_____

_____

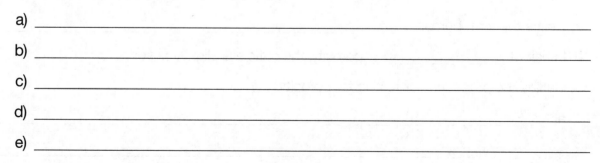

Understand Why People Color Their Hair

3. Identify the common reasons why people color their hair.

a) _____

b) _____

c) _____

d) _____

e) _____

Review Hair Facts

4. The structure of the client's hair and the desired results determine which haircolor to use.

_____ True   _____ False

Rationale:

5. Name the three major components of hair.

1) _____

2) _____

3) _____

6. The _____, the middle layer of hair, gives the hair the majority of its strength and elasticity.

7. In hair, melanin is distributed evenly regardless of texture.

_____ True   _____ False

Rationale:

8. Hair _____, the number of hairs per square inch, can range from thin to thick.

9. Define the term porosity. _____

10. In hair of _____ porosity, the cuticle is slightly raised.

11. Outline the procedure for testing for porosity.

a) _____

_____

_____

b) _____

_____

_____

c) _____

_____

_____

Identify Natural Hair Color and Tone

12. List the three types of melanin in the cortex.

1) _____

2) _____

3) _____

13. _____, also known as undertone, is the varying degrees of warmth exposed during a permanent color or lightening process.

14. _____ is the unit of measurement used to identify the lightness or darkness of a color.

15. Haircolor levels are arranged on a scale of 1 to 10, with _____ being the darkest and _____ the lightest.

16. The first step when performing a haircolor service is to _____ _____.

17. What are the four steps to determining natural level?

1) _____

_____

_____

_____

2) _____

_____

_____

_____

3) _____

_____

_____

_____

4) _____

_____

_____

_____

18. A(n) _____ is the predominant tone of a color.

19. Equal parts of blue and yellow always make green.

_____ True   _____ False

Rationale:

20. _____ colors are pure or fundamental colors that cannot be created by combining other colors.

21. Which of the following is the weakest of the primary colors?

_____ a) Yellow   _____ c) Red

_____ b) Blue   _____ d) Orange

22. When all three primary colors are present in equal proportions, the resulting color is _____.

23. Black can be used to deepen a color.

_____ True   _____ False

Rationale:

24. Which of the following is a secondary color?

_____ a) Red   _____ c) Green

_____ b) Yellow   _____ d) Blue

25. Complementary colors neutralize each other.

_____ True   _____ False

Rationale:

26. The stylist should use which of the following colors to neutralize orange?

_____ a) Yellow   _____ c) Blue

_____ b) Violet   _____ d) Green

27. Name the four warm tones that can look lighter than their actual levels.

1) _____

2) _____

3) _____

4) _____

28. _____ refers to the strength of a color.

Understand the Types of Haircolor

29. Identify the two categories of haircoloring products.

1) _____

2) _____

30. Which of the following is a use of demipermanent color?

_____ a) Adds subtle results   _____ c) Creates bright changes

_____ b) Blends gray hair   _____ d) Covers grey

31. List the roles of an alkalizing ingredient.

a) _____

b) _____

c) _____

32. The pigments in temporary color penetrate the cuticle layer.

_____ True   _____ False

> Rationale:

33. Traditional semipermanent haircolor lasts _____ to _____ weeks, depending on how frequently the hair is shampooed.

34. Why are demipermanent haircolor products able to deposit without lifting?

_____

_____

_____

35. Permanent haircoloring products are regarded as the best products for covering gray hair.

_____ True   _____ False

> Rationale:

36. Metallic haircolors are known as _____ colors.

37. Henna is usually available only in what tones?

_____

38. Metallic haircolors require frequent applications and historically have been marketed to women.

_____ True   _____ False

> Rationale:

39. A(n) _____ is an oxidizing agent that, when mixed with an oxidation haircolor, supplies the necessary oxygen gas to develop the color molecules and create a change in natural hair color.

40. What volume hydrogen peroxide should you use with high-lift colors?

_____ a) 10   _____ c) 30

_____ b) 20   _____ d) 40

41. List the objectives of hair lighteners.

a) _____

b) _____

c) _____

d) _____

e) _____

f) _____

g) _____

42. During the process of decolorizing, natural hair can go through as many as
_____ stages.

43. How are toners used?

_____

_____

Conduct an Effective Haircolor Consultation

44. A haircolor consultation is the most critical part of the color service.

_____ True   _____ False

Rationale:

45. Medications can affect hair color.

_____ True   _____ False

Rationale:

46. Give some examples of leading questions to ask during the consultation.

a) _____

_____

b) _____

_____

c) _____

_____

d) _____

_____

e) _____

_____

f) _____

_____

g) _____

_____

h) _____

_____

i) _____

_____

j) _____

_____

47. What is the purpose of the release statement?

_____

_____

_____

_____

_____

Formulate Haircolor

48. List the five basic questions you should always ask when formulating a haircolor.

1) _____

2) _____

3) _____

4) _____

5) _____

49. Permanent color is applied by what two methods?

1) _____

2) _____

50. A patch test must be given _____ to _____ hours before the application of any aniline haircolor.

51. Give the procedure for performing a patch test.

a) _____

_____

b) _____

_____

c) _____

_____

d) _____

_____

e) _____

_____

f) _____

_____

g) _____

_____

Apply Haircolor

52. The strand test is performed before the client is prepared for the coloring service.

_____ True   _____ False

Rationale:

53. Name the materials, implements, and supplies needed for temporary haircolor application.

a) _____

b) _____

c) _____

d) _____

e) _____

f) _____

g) _____

h) _____

i) _____

54. Semipermanent colors only deposit color.

_____ True   _____ False

Rationale:

55. The application procedure for demipermanent haircolor is similar to that of a traditional semipermanent color.

_____ True   _____ False

Rationale:

56. In a(n) _____ application, hair is colored for the first time.

57. When lightening a virgin head of hair, how far away from the scalp should the lightener be applied? _____

58. Outline the procedure for permanent single-process retouch with a glaze.

a) _____

b) _____

c) _____

d) _____

_____

_____

_____

_____

_____

e) _____

_____

f) _____

_____

g) _____

h) _____

59. What is the purpose of double-process, high-lift coloring?

_____

_____

Show How to Use Lighteners

60. Colorists can choose from what three forms of lightener?

1) _____

2) _____

3) _____

61. Name the features and benefits of cream lighteners.

a) _____

_____

_____

b) _____

_____

_____

c) _____

_____

_____

62. _____ are powdered persulfate salts added to haircolor to increase its lightening ability.

63. Discuss the use of powdered off-the-scalp lighteners.

_____

_____

_____

_____

64. Why is a preliminary strand test performed?

_____

_____

_____

_____

65. Compare the procedure for a lightener retouch with that for lightening a virgin head of hair.

_____

_____

_____

Express How to Use Toners

66. Toners require a double-process application.

_____ True _____ False

Rationale:

67. Detail the procedure for toner application. The first and last steps have been provided to help you get started.

a) Pre-lighten the hair to the desired stage of decolorization.

b) _____

c) _____

d) _____

e) _____

f) _____

g) _____
_____

h) _____
_____

i) _____
_____
_____
_____

j) _____
_____

k) _____
_____

l) _____

_____

m) _____

n) _____

o) _____

_____

p) _____

q) Style as desired. Use caution to avoid stretching the hair.

Create Special Effects Using Haircoloring Techniques

68. _____, also known as lowlighting, is the technique of coloring strands of hair darker than the natural color.

69. What are the three most common methods for achieving highlights?

1) _____

2) _____

3) _____

70. In the procedure for special effects haircoloring with foil, start by dividing the hair into _____ quadrants.

71. The _____ technique, also known as the free-form technique, involves the painting of a lightener (usually powdered off-the-scalp lightener) directly onto clean, styled hair.

72. When are highlighting shampoos used?

_____

_____

Understand the Special Challenges in Haircolor and Corrective Solutions

73. Name the factors that can develop a yellow cast in gray hair.

a) _____

b) _____

c) _____

d) _____

74. For gray hair, formulations from level _____ will provide better coverage and can be used to create pastel and blond tones if desired.

75. For hair that is 30 to 50 percent gray, the semipermanent/demipermanent color formulation should be:

_____ a) One level lighter than the desired level

_____ b) Two levels lighter than the desired level

_____ c) Equal parts one and two levels lighter

_____ d) Equal parts desired and one level lighter

76. Give tips for achieving gray coverage.

a) _____

b) _____

c) _____

d) _____

e) _____

f) _____

g) _____

77. _____ is the process of treating gray or very resistant hair to allow for better penetration of color.

78. List guidelines for effective color correction.

a) _____

b) _____

c) _____

d) _____

e) _____

f) _____

g) _____

79. List the characteristics of damaged hair.

a) _____

b) _____

c) _____

d) _____

e) _____

f) _____

g) _____

80. _____ fillers are used to recondition damaged, overly porous hair and equalize porosity so that the hair accepts the color evenly from strand to strand and from scalp to ends, while _____ fillers equalize porosity and deposit color in one application to provide a uniform contributing pigment on pre-lightened hair.

81. Yellow blond hair can be corrected to a natural blond by adding what two colors?

1) _____

2) _____

82. Fading is uncommon with color-treated red hair.

_____ True   _____ False

Rationale:

83. List haircolor tips for redheads.

a) _____

_____

b) _____

_____

c) _____

_____

d) _____

_____

e) _____

_____

_____

84. What are some haircolor tips for blonds?

a) _____

_____

b) _____

_____

c) _____

d) _____

_____

e) _____

_____

_____

_____

_____

_____

85. What is the solution for hair with a green cast?

_____

_____

_____

_____

86. What should the stylist do if the overall hair color is too dark?

_____

_____

_____

_____

_____

87. Provide the steps for restoring blond hair to its natural color.

a) _____

_____

_____

_____

_____

_____

b) _____

_____

_____

_____

_____

c) _____

_____

_____

_____

_____

_____

_____

88. **ACTIVITY:** Work with a fellow student for this partner activity. Each using your mannequin, section the hair into four quadrants by parting from the center of the front hairline to the center of the nape, and from the top of one ear to the top of the other ear. Now the fun begins. Each student in the pair should create a different color mistake in each quadrant. Once the colors have been processed, shampooed, conditioned, and rinsed, record the formulas and timing used in each quadrant as you would a client service record card. Now, exchange mannequins and, using the haircoloring knowledge you gained in this chapter and the information contained in the client service record

card, correct the mistakes you each made on your respective mannequins. Record your results on the client service record card. Be prepared to explain your results to the instructor, whether the corrective actions were satisfactory or not.

_____

_____

_____

Know Haircoloring Safety Precautions

89. List haircoloring safety precautions. The first precaution is provided to help you get started.

a) Perform a patch test 24 to 48 hours before each application of aniline-derivative haircolor. Apply haircolor only if the patch test is negative.

b) _____

c) _____

d) _____

e) _____

f) _____

g) _____

h) _____

i) _____

j) _____

k) _____

l) _____

m) _____

n) _____

o) _____

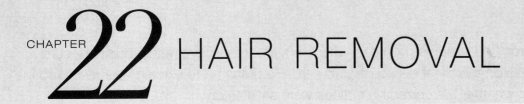

Date: _____

Rating: _____

Text Pages: 736–763

1. Hair removal is one of the fastest growing services in the salon and spa business.

   _____ True   _____ False

Rationale:

2. The most common form of hair removal in salons and spas is _____ .

3. Many men are now requesting hair removal services.

   _____ True   _____ False

Rationale:

4. Check the most frequent hair removal requests for men in the list below.

   _____ a) Nape of the neck   _____ d) Feet

   _____ b) Chest   _____ e) Nose

   _____ c) Back

5. _____, also known as _____, refers to the growth of an unusual amount of hair on parts of the body normally bearing only downy hair, such as the faces of women or the backs of men.

6. Name the two major categories of hair removal.

   1) _____

   2) _____

why study HAIR REMOVAL?

7. In your own words, explain why cosmetologists should study and thoroughly understand hair removal.

   _____

   _____

   _____

   _____

   _____

   _____

   _____

   _____

Consult the Client

8. The _____ is a questionnaire that discloses all medications, both topical and oral, along with any known medical issues, skin disorders, or allergies that might affect treatment.

9. List some medications that may render a client unsuited to hair removal services.

   a) _____

   b) _____

   c) _____

   d) _____

   e) _____

10. How often should clients complete release forms for hair removal services?

   _____ a) Prior to every service   _____ c) Every year

   _____ b) Every other visit   _____ d) Once at initial visit

Name the Contraindications for Hair Removal

11. Waxing or hair removal should not be performed anywhere on the body of clients to whom any of the following situations apply. The first situation has been provided to help you get started.

a) Client has used isotretinoin (Accutane) in the last six months.

b) _____

_____

c) _____

_____

d) _____

_____

e) _____

_____

f) _____

_____

g) _____

_____

h) _____

_____

i) _____

_____

j) _____

_____

k) _____

_____

l) _____

_____

m) _____

_____

12. Facial waxing should not be performed on clients with any of the following conditions without first obtaining permission from their physician:

a) _____

_____

b) _____

_____

c) _____

_____

d) _____

_____

e) _____

_____

f) _____

_____

g) _____

_____

Describe Permanent Hair Removal

13. Match each of the following types of permanent hair removal with its definition.

_____ Electrolysis   a) Technique that uses intense light to destroy the growth cells of the hair follicles

_____ Photoepilation   b) Method in which a beam pulses on the skin, impairing hair growth

_____ Laser hair removal   c) Removal of hair by means of an electric current that destroys the growth cells of hair

14. Who can perform electrolysis?

_____

15. Who can perform photoepilation?

_____

_____

16. Clinical studies have shown that photoepilation can provide _____ to _____ percent clearance of hair in _____ weeks.

17. Laser hair removal is most effective when used on follicles in the _____ or _____ phase.

18. What type of hair responds best to laser treatment?

_____

19. Is laser hair removal permanent?

_____

_____

20. Who can perform laser hair removal?

_____

_____

Discuss Temporary Hair Removal

21. Name the methods of temporary hair removal.

a) _____

b) _____

c) _____

d) _____

e) _____

f) _____

22. _____ is the most common form of temporary hair removal, particularly of men's facial hair.

23. Prior to shaving, a _____ can help reduce irritation.

24. _____ is commonly used to shape the eyebrows and remove undesirable hairs from around the mouth and chin.

25. The natural arch of the eyebrow follows the _____, or the curved line of the eye socket.

26. Explain how to determine the best shape for an eyebrow.

_____

_____

_____

_____

_____

_____

_____

27. A(n) _____ is a substance, usually a caustic alkali preparation, used for the temporary removal of superfluous hair by dissolving it at the skin's surface.

28. What happens when a depilatory is applied?

_____

_____

29. It is a good idea to patch test any depilatory on the client's skin prior to treatment for the first time.

_____ True   _____ False

Rationale:

30. Which of the following is considered inappropriate for temporary hair removal from the arms?

_____ a) Waxing   _____ b) Tweezing   _____ c) Depilatories

31. A(n) _____ removes hair from the bottom of the follicle.

32. Wax is a commonly used epilator.

_____ True _____ False

Rationale:

33. The time between waxings is generally _____ to _____ weeks.

34. Wax may be applied to various parts of the face and body, such as the

_____, _____, _____,

_____, _____, and _____.

35. For a waxing service, hair should be at least _____ long, but no longer than _____.

36. _____ is a waxing technique that requires the removal of all hair from the front and the back of the bikini area.

37. Removing _____ or _____ hair may cause the skin to temporarily feel less soft.

38. Before beginning a wax treatment, be sure the client completes a _____ and signs a(n) _____.

39. Why should disposable gloves be worn during waxing?

_____

_____

40. List the implements, materials, and supplies needed for an eyebrow waxing using soft wax. The first two items have been provided to help you get started.

a) Brow brush.

b) Cotton pads and swabs.

c) _____

d) _____

e) _____

f) _____

g) _____

h) _____

i) _____

j) _____

k) _____

l) _____

m) _____

n) _____

o) _____

41. (W) **ACTIVITY:** In the chart below, place the steps of the Lip Waxing Using Hard Wax procedure in the proper order.

Step Number	Action
	Lay a clean towel over the top of the facial chair and then a layer of disposable paper.
	Allow the wax to sit for 1 to 2 minutes. Using your index finger and thumb, gently lift the edge of the wax and pull off the wax in an upwards and inwards movement.
	Determine which technique for applying hard wax over the lip is to be performed.
	Cleanse the skin with a mild emollient cleanser and apply an emollient or antiseptic lotion.
	Remove client's makeup, cleanse the area thoroughly with a mild cleanser, and dry.
	Melt the wax in the heater.
	Remove any remaining wax residue from the skin with a gentle wax remover.
	Test the temperature and consistency of the heated wax.
	With spatula or applicator, apply the warmed hard wax to the skin over the lip evenly from center of lip towards the corner of mouth in the same direction of the hair growth, about the thickness of a nickel.
	Repeat the application and removal in the same manner on the other side of the lip.
	Put on disposable gloves.
	Immediately apply pressure to the waxed area with your finger. Hold your finger for approximately 5 seconds to relieve discomfort.
	With the spatula or applicator, first apply the warmed, hard wax about the thickness of a nickel to the skin in the opposite direction of hair growth.
	Place a hair cap or headband on the client's head to keep hair away from the face.

42. Explain how to apply soft wax in the body waxing procedure.

_____

_____

_____

_____

_____

43. _____ is a temporary hair removal method whereby cotton thread is twisted and rolled along the surface of the skin, entwining the hair in the thread and lifting it from the follicle.

44. Sugaring produces the same results as soft or hard wax.

_____ True   _____ False

Rationale:

45. After sugaring, residue can be removed from the skin by dissolving it with

_____.

46. List the steps in the pre-service procedure for preparing a treatment room.

a) _____

_____

b) _____

_____

c) _____

_____

d) _____

_____

e) _____

_____

f) _____

_____

_____

_____

g) _____

_____

_____

_____

_____

_____

_____

h) _____

_____

_____

_____

i) _____

_____

_____

_____

47. Give the steps to follow at the end of each day with respect to the treatment room. The first step has been provided to help you get started.

a) Put on a fresh pair of gloves to protect yourself from contact with soiled linens and implements.

b) _____

_____

_____

c) _____

_____

_____

d) _____

_____

_____

e) _____

_____

_____

f) _____

_____

_____

g) _____

_____

_____

h) _____

_____

_____

i) _____

_____

_____

j) _____

_____

_____

k) _____

_____

_____

l) _____

_____

_____

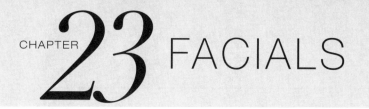

Date: _____

Rating: _____

Text Pages: 764–809

1. Facial treatments can be very relaxing and offer many improvements to the _____ of the skin.

2. Proper skin care can make oily skin look _____, dry skin look and feel more _____, and aging skin look _____ _____.

why study FACIALS?

3. In your own words, explain why cosmetologists should study and thoroughly understand facials.

_____

_____

_____

_____

_____

_____

_____

_____

_____

_____

Conduct a Consultation and Skin Analysis

4. The opportunity to ask clients questions about their health and skin care history and to advise them about appropriate home-care products and treatments comes during the _____.

5. Explain the importance of skin analysis.

_____

_____

_____

6. What is the main purpose of the client intake form?

_____

_____

7. A(n) _____ is a condition that requires avoiding certain treatments, procedures, or products to prevent undesirable side effects.

8. Name the main contraindications to look for. The first contraindication to look for has been provided to help you get started.

a) Use of isotretinoin (Accutane).

b) _____

c) _____

d) _____

e) _____

f) _____

g) _____

h) _____

i) _____

j) _____

k) _____

l) _____

m) _____

n) _____

9. Clients with obvious skin abnormalities or other abnormal-looking signs should be referred to a physician for treatment.

_____ True   _____ False

Rationale:

10. What information is obtained via the client intake form that can be transcribed onto the service record card?

a) _____

_____

_____

b) _____

_____

_____

c) _____

_____

_____

d) _____

_____

_____

e) _____

_____

_____

f) _____

_____

_____

g) _____

_____

_____

h) _____

_____

_____

i) _____

_____

_____

Determine Skin Type During the Skin Analysis

11. Normal skin is very unusual.

_____ True   _____ False

Rationale:

12. Which of the following skin types has obvious pores down the center of the face?

_____ a) Combination oily   _____ c) Combination dry

_____ b) Acne   _____ d) Oily

13. Obvious, large pores indicate _____ skin, lack of visible pores indicates _____ skin.

14. Cosmetologists should avoid wearing jewelry on the hands or arms while administering

facial treatments because _____

_____.

15. _____ is determined by how oily or dry the skin is.

16. Skin type can be permanently changed by treatment.

_____ True   _____ False

Rationale:

17. The amount of sebum produced by the _____ determines the size of the pores and is _____.

18. The term *alipidic* means _____, and describes skin that does not produce enough sebum.

19. Oily skin that produces too much sebum will have _____, and the skin may appear to be _____.

20. Describe open comedones.

_____

_____

21. Define closed comedones.

_____

_____

22. Why is acne considered a skin type?

_____

_____

23. Acne bacteria are anaerobic, which means _____

_____.

24. Conditions of the skin are generally treatable.

_____ True   _____ False

Rationale:

25. Describe what dehydration looks like.

_____

_____

_____

26. List some causes of dehydration.

a) _____

b) _____

c) _____

27. How is dehydrated skin treated?

_____

_____

_____

28. Describe hyperpigmentation.

_____

_____

_____

29. How is hyperpigmentation treated?

_____

_____

_____

30. Explain how to identify sensitive skin.

_____

_____

_____

31. What should you avoid when treating sensitive skin?

_____

_____

32. _____ is a chronic hereditary disorder that can be indicated by constant or frequent facial blushing.

33. _____ are distended or dilated surface blood vessels, while _____ are areas of skin with distended capillaries and diffuse redness.

Aging and Sun-Damaged Skin

34. Describe aging skin.

_____

_____

35. How is aging skin treated?

_____

_____

36. Describe sun-damaged skin.

_____

_____

_____

_____

_____

Categorize Skin Care Products

37. Name the two types of cleanser.

    1) _____

    2) _____

38. Toners, also known as _____ or _____, are lotions that help rebalance the pH and remove remnants of cleanser from the skin.

39. Exfoliants can improve the appearance of wrinkles, aging, and hyperpigmentation.

    _____ True   _____ False

Rationale:

40. _____, also called roll-off masks, are peeling creams that are rubbed off of the skin.

41. Discuss the use of alpha hydroxy acids.

_____

_____

_____

_____

_____

_____

42. Compare the two basic types of keratolytic enzyme peels.

_____

_____

_____

_____

_____

_____

43. Name some ways in which exfoliation improves the skin's appearance.

a) _____

b) _____

c) _____

d) _____

e) _____

f) _____

g) _____

44. Oily skin does not need much emollient.

_____ True   _____ False

Rationale:

45. Shielding the skin from sun exposure is probably the most important habit to benefit the skin.

_____ True   _____ False

Rationale:

46. _____ are individual doses of serum, sealed in small vials.

47. Cream masks do not dry on the skin like clay masks do and are often used to moisturize dry skin.

_____ True   _____ False

Rationale:

48. Discuss the preparation and application of modelage masks.

_____

_____

_____

_____

_____

_____

49. Describe the use of gauze for mask application.

_____

_____

_____

_____

_____

_____

Learn the Basic Techniques of a Facial Massage

50. _____ is the manual or mechanical manipulation of the body by rubbing, gently pinching, kneading, tapping, and using other movements to increase metabolism and circulation, to promote absorption, and to relieve pain.

51. In facial massage, the direction of movement is always _____

_____.

52. Describe effleurage.

_____

_____

53. Pressure is a key component of effleurage.

_____ True   _____ False

Rationale:

54. Describe pétrissage.

_____

_____

55. Fulling is used mainly for massaging the _____.

56. List and describe the variations of friction.

a) _____

_____

_____

b) _____

_____

_____

c) _____

_____

_____

57. Tapotement is the most stimulating form of massage.

_____ True   _____ False

Rationale:

58. Name the body parts on which hacking is used.

a) _____

b) _____

c) _____

59. Vibration should be applied at the _____ of a massage.

60. Every muscle has a _____, which is a point on the skin that covers the muscle where pressure or stimulation will cause contraction of that muscle.

61. Name the benefits of proper face and scalp massage.

a) _____

b) _____

c) _____

d) _____

e) _____

f) _____

g) _____

62. How does a cosmetologist perform linear movement over the forehead?

_____

_____

_____

63. What facial movement does the accompanying figure illustrate?

_____

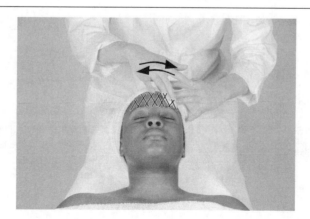

64. Explain how to perform the light tapping movement.

_____

_____

_____

65. Describe how to perform the chest and back movement.

_____

_____

_____

Know the Purpose of the Facial Equipment

66. A facial _____ heats and produces a stream of warm steam that can be focused on the client's face or other areas of skin.

67. _____ brushes are used for back treatment, while _____ brushes are used for the face.

How Electrotherapy and Light Therapy Treat the Skin

68. Identify the contraindications of electrotherapy.

_____

_____

_____

_____

69. Galvanic machines have two positive electrodes called a(n) _____, which has a red plug and cord, and a negative electrode called a(n) _____, which has a black plug and cord.

70. Desincrustation is very helpful when treating oily areas with multiple comedones and most acne-prone skin.

_____ True   _____ False

Rationale:

71. _____ is the process of using galvanic current to enable water-soluble products that contain ions to penetrate the skin.

72. Microcurrent is best known for helping to tone the skin, producing a lifting effect for aging skin that lacks elasticity.

_____ a) True   _____ b) False

Rationale:

73. Explain direct and indirect application of high-frequency current.

_____

_____

_____

_____

74. Explain the use of light-emitting diode (LED) treatment in cosmetology.

_____

_____

_____

_____

_____

_____

75. _____ is a type of mechanical exfoliation that involves shooting aluminum oxide or other crystals at the skin with a hand-held device that exfoliates dead cells.

Use Facials to Treat Basic and Specialty Skin Types

76. Facial treatments fall into what two categories?

1) _____

2) _____

77. A preservative treatment is meant to _____

_____

_____.

78. A corrective treatment is meant to _____

_____.

79. What are the guidelines for performing a facial treatment?

a) _____

_____

b) _____

_____

c) _____

_____

d) _____

_____

e) _____

_____

f) _____

_____

g) _____

_____

h) _____

_____

80. How should the client prepare for a basic facial?

_____

_____

81. Where should the client change prior to the facial?

_____

82. Give the procedure for draping the client's hair for a basic facial.

a) _____

_____

_____

b) _____

_____

_____

c) _____

_____

_____

83. Discuss how to steam a client's face for a basic facial.

_____

_____

_____

_____

84. What is the proper procedure for applying a treatment mask during a basic facial?

a) _____

_____

b) _____

_____

c) _____

_____

_____

85. How is the treatment mask removed during a basic facial?

_____

_____

86. After the treatment mask is removed during a basic facial, what should be applied?

_____

_____

87. List the steps in the procedure for a dry skin facial that follow the proper pre-service, draping, removal of client makeup, skin analysis, and cleansing steps. The first and last steps are listed to help you get started. Assume you are *not* using electrotherapy.

a) Focus steam on the face and allow steaming for 5 minutes.

b) _____

_____

_____

c) _____

_____

_____

d) _____

_____

_____

e) _____

_____

_____

f) _____

_____

_____

g) _____

_____

_____

h) _____

_____

_____

i) _____

_____

_____

j) _____

_____

_____

k) _____

_____

_____

l) _____

_____

_____

m) When the service is completed, remove the head covering and show the client to the dressing room, offering assistance if needed.

88. In addition to the items needed for a basic facial, what items are needed for a facial on oily skin with open comedones?

a) _____

b) _____

c) _____

89. Minor problem skin and oily skin respond poorly to facial treatments.

_____ True   _____ False

Rationale:

90. When treating acne-prone skin, disposable gloves should be worn throughout the treatment.

_____ True   _____ False

Rationale:

91. How can cosmetologists help clients with acne-prone skin?

_____

_____

_____

92. Acne-prone skin should not be massaged.

_____ True   _____ False

Rationale:

93. After extraction is complete in a facial for acne-prone and problem skin, what steps must the cosmetologist complete?

a) _____

_____

_____

b) _____

_____

_____

c) _____

_____

_____

d) _____

_____

_____

e) _____

_____

_____

f) _____

_____

_____

g) _____

_____

_____

h) _____

_____

_____

i) _____

_____

_____

j) _____

_____

_____

94. Home care is probably the most important factor in a successful skin care program.

_____ True   _____ False

Rationale:

95. 🖐 **ACTIVITY:** You have learned in this chapter how facial steaming can be effective in opening pores, stimulating circulation, and helping masks and creams work more effectively. Effective steaming does not require expensive machines or equipment. It can be successfully accomplished in your own home. Consider this: Pull your hair back and secure it before cleansing and washing your face thoroughly. Prepare a 2-quart saucepan with water and add herbs such as peppermint, eucalyptus, chamomile, and lavender, which all disinfect and soothe the skin. Ingredients such as lemon juice and sage can also be effective. Bring the ingredients to a boil and place the pan on a table or countertop. Lower your cleansed face above the pan and drape a towel over your head and around the pan to minimize the escape of steam. Allow your face to enjoy the steam for no longer than 10 minutes. Upon completion, blot your face with a soft towel. Your skin is now prepared for a mask or exfoliation treatment. If you do not wish

to continue with these additional treatments, refresh the skin with cool water to close the pores. Below, record the ingredients you used in your personal steaming formula. Explain how your skin felt after the exercise and what you might do differently next time.

Use of Aromatherapy in the Basic Facial

96. The therapeutic use of plant aromas for beauty and health treatment is known as
_____.

97. Cosmetologists are qualified to perform healing treatments with aromatherapy.

_____ True   _____ False

Rationale:

24 FACIAL MAKEUP

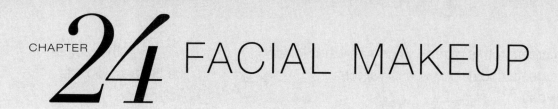

Date: _____

Rating: _____

Text Pages: 810–845

1. Makeup artistry is a very rewarding segment of cosmetology that produces _____ results that alter how clients view themselves.

why study FACIAL MAKEUP?

2. In your own words, explain why cosmetologists should study and thoroughly understand facial makeup.

_____

_____

_____

_____

_____

_____

_____

_____

Describe Facial Makeup and Their Uses

3. List the forms of foundation.

a) _____

b) _____

c) _____

d) _____

4. _____ were created to actually neutralize skin discolorations.

5. Liquid and cream forms of makeup are an emulsion of _____ that act as spreading agents and help suspend various _____ like titanium dioxide and iron oxides.

6. Often a foundation will contain aluminum or some other drying agent to help the product set quickly when applied to the skin to produce a _____, non-shiny finish.

7. _____ foundation, also known as _____, is considerably thicker than a liquid.

8. Cosmetic products that do not contain ingredients that clog the follicles are called _____.

9. Match each of the following cosmetics with their function or description.

Cosmetic		**Function**
_____ Concealer	a)	Heavy makeup used for theatrical purposes
_____ Face powder	b)	Defines the shape of the lips
_____ Eye shadow	c)	Also known as blush
_____ Eyeliner	d)	Accentuates the eye shape
_____ Eyebrow pencils	e)	Makes lash line appear fuller
_____ Cheek color	f)	Contains solvents
_____ Lip color	g)	Heavy-coverage pressed powder
_____ Lip liner	h)	Hides dark eye circles and hyperpigmentation
_____ Mascara	i)	Creates a matte or non-shiny finish
_____ Eye makeup remover	j)	Adds color and shape to eyebrows
_____ Greasepaint	k)	Used to darken, define, and thicken the eyelashes
_____ Cake makeup	l)	Enhances the lips

10. Match each of the following makeup implements with its use.

_____ Powder brush	a)	Removes excess facial hair
_____ Blush brush	b)	Applies powder to the eyebrows or eye liner at the lash line
_____ Concealer brush	c)	Applies powder cheek color
_____ Lip brush	d)	Diffuses and blends shadow
_____ Eye shadow brush	e)	Lifts and curls the upper lashes

_____ Eyeliner brush   f) Separates eyelashes after mascara application

_____ Angle brush   g) Applies concealer around the eyes and cover
                                   blemishes

_____ Lash comb   h) Applies powder

_____ Brow bush (spoolie)   i) Applies liquid liner or shadow to the lash line

_____ Tweezers   j) Applies lip color

_____ Eyelash curler   k) Applies mascara to the lashes or brush brows
                                   into place

11. What can be used to quickly clean brushes, although due to the high level of alcohol
    content, they are not recommended for daily use?

    _____

12. Single-use implements are disposable and should be discarded after one use. List
    below the single-use items used in makeup applications. The first implement is provided
    to help you get started.

    a) Sponges.

    b) _____

    c) _____

    d) _____

    e) _____

    f) _____

    g) _____

    h) _____

How to Use Color Theory for Makeup Application

13. Identify the three main factors to consider when choosing colors for a client.

    1) _____

    2) _____

    3) _____

14. _____ colors range from yellow and gold to orange, red-orange, most
    reds, and even some yellow-greens. _____ colors encompass blues,
    greens, violets, and blue-reds.

15. When choosing colors for clients, pairing warm and cool colors is recommended.

_____ True _____ False

Rationale:

16. Pale peach is a warm color for which of the following skin tones?

_____ a) Fair _____ b) Medium _____ c) Dark

17. A neutral skin tone contains equal elements of warm and cool, no matter how fair or deep the skin is.

_____ True _____ False

Rationale:

18. Matching eye shadow with eye color is the best way to create dramatic depth of contrast.

_____ True _____ False

Rationale:

19. _____ is the complementary color to blue eyes. Red is the complementary color to _____ eyes. _____ eyes are neutral and can wear any color.

20. The cosmetologist should coordinate cheek and lip makeup in the same color family as eye makeup.

_____ True _____ False

Rationale:

21. _____ color needs to be taken into account when determining eye makeup color.

22. Blue is a cool color for which of the following hair colors?

_____ a) Blonde   _____ c) Brown

_____ b) Red   _____ d) Black

23. Skin primers are applied after any colored foundation.

_____ True   _____ False

Rationale:

Alter Face Shapes with Makeup

24. The basic rule when altering a face shape is that drawing light to an area _____ features, while creating a shadow _____ them.

25. A _____ is formed when a product that is darker than the client's skin tone is used to create shadows over _____ features so they are less noticeable.

26. The oval-shaped face is divided into three equal _____ sections. The first third is measured from the _____. The second third is measured from the _____. The last third is measured from the _____.

27. The oval face is approximately _____ as wide as it is long.

28. The ideal distance between the eyes is the width of _____.

29. The round face is usually broader in proportion to its length than the oval face.

_____ True   _____ False

Rationale:

30. The _____ face is composed of comparatively straight lines with a wide forehead and square jawline.

31. A jawline that is wider than the forehead characterizes the _____ face.

32. The _____, or heart-shaped face, has a wide forehead, narrow jawline, and pointed chin.

33. The _____ face has a narrow forehead with the greatest width across the cheekbones.

34. The _____ face has greater length in proportion to its width than the square or round face.

35. For a _____ forehead, applying a lighter foundation just above the brows broadens the appearance.

36. For a _____ forehead, applying a darker foundation over the prominent area minimizes the forehead.

37. For a _____ nose, apply a darker foundation along the sides of the nose.

38. If the nostrils are wide, apply a _____ foundation to both sides of the nostrils.

39. For a broad nose, use a _____ foundation along the sides of the nose and nostrils.

40. To balance a _____ chin and receding nose, shadow the tip of the chin with a darker foundation and highlight the bridge of the nose with a lighter foundation.

41. For a(n) _____ chin, highlight the chin by using a lighter foundation than the one used on the face.

42. For a(n) _____ chin, use a darker foundation on the sagging portion, and use a natural skin tone foundation on the face.

43. To correct a(n) _____ jawline, highlight the thinnest areas with a lighter shade of foundation.

44. _____ eyes can be lengthened by extending the shadow beyond the outer corner of the eyes.

45. _____ eyes are closer together than the width of one eye.

46. For eyes that are too close together, create space by applying a thin layer of light concealer to _____, near the bridge of the nose.

47. _____ eyes can be minimized by blending the deeper color shadow over the prominent part of the upper lid.

48. For _____, lift the lid at the brow to reveal the natural contours. Apply a slightly deeper shadow through the crease. Blend to minimize any hard lines and create a natural look.

49. For _____ eyes, apply the shadow from the inner corners of the eyebrows toward the nose, and blend carefully.

50. For _____ eyes, use bright, light, reflective colors. Create a wash of color across the lid. Use a light-to-medium color along the lash line and outer corners of the eyes.

51. For _____ under eyes, apply a color correcting concealer over the area to neutralize discoloration. Blend and smooth the product into the surrounding area. Set lightly with translucent powder.

52. _____ eyebrows can make the face look puffy or protruding, or may give the eyes a surprised look.

53. The ideal eyebrow shape is positioned along three lines. The first line runs vertically, from the _____ upward.

54. The second line to determine the ideal eyebrow shape runs from the _____ _____ upward. This is where the highest part of the arch should be.

55. The third line of the ideal eyebrow shape is drawn at an angle from the _____ _____.

56. What should you do if the eyebrow arch is too high?

_____

_____

_____

57. People with low foreheads should have a _____ to their eyebrow shape, which gives more height to a very low forehead.

58. If a person has _____ eyes, build up the inside corners of the eyebrows.

59. If a person has _____ eyes, widen the distance between the eyebrows and slightly extend them outward.

60. If a person has a round face, arch the brows _____ to make the face appear narrower.

61. If a person has a long face, making the eyebrows almost _____ can create the illusion of a shorter face.

62. If a person has a square face, the face will appear more oval if there is a(n) _____ arch on the ends of the eyebrows.

63. _____ are lash lengtheners that contain fibers to make lashes look longer and fuller.

64. Lips are usually positioned so that the peaks of the upper lip fall directly in line with the nostrils.

_____ True   _____ False

Rationale:

65. What can you do for a client who has ruddy skin?

_____

_____

66. What can you do for a client who has sallow skin?

_____

_____

67. A corrective makeup technique used to conceal scars, burns, and pigmentation issues ranging from vitiligo to tattoos is called _____.

Outline the Steps for Basic Makeup Application

68. Artificial lighting is the first and best choice for makeup consultations.

_____ True   _____ False

Rationale:

69. What is the role of a client instruction sheet?

_____

_____

_____

70. Explain how to choose the correct foundation color.

_____

_____

_____

71. A(n) _____ is an obvious line where foundation begins and ends.

72. Contrast how the different types of foundation are applied.

_____

_____

_____

73. Explain how to apply concealer.

_____

_____

_____

_____

_____

74. A concealer may be worn alone, without foundation, if chosen and blended correctly.

_____ True   _____ False

Rationale:

75. Describe how loose face powder is applied.

_____

_____

_____

_____

_____

76. How are eyebrow pencils used?

_____

_____

_____

_____

77. What should be done with the eyeliner pencil before each use?

_____

78. To apply powder eye shadow, scrape the product onto a palette or tissue with a
spatula, and then use an applicator or clean brush. Then simply apply the color close
to the _____.
Blend to achieve the desired effect.

79. Which finger is used to dab cream eye shadow onto the center of the eyelid?

_____.

80. What eyeliner color do most clients prefer?

_____

81. Powder blush should be applied in a circle on the apple of the cheek, beyond the
corner of the eye, or inward between the cheekbone and the nose.

_____ True   _____ False

Rationale:

82. _____ blush is applied after the foundation and before powder so that it
blends into the foundation.

83. After lip color has been removed from the container, how is it applied?

_____

_____

_____

_____

_____

_____

_____

84. Mascara may be used on all lashes, both _____.

85. When applying mascara, it is okay to double dip the wand.

_____ True   _____ False

Rationale:

86. When using an eyelash curler, when should you curl the lashes?

_____

Apply Artificial Eyelashes

87. _____ are eyelash hairs on a band that are applied with adhesive to the natural lash line.

88. _____ are separate artificial eyelashes that are applied to the base of the eyelashes one at a time.

89. List the implements and materials needed to apply false eyelashes. The first item has been provided to get you started.

a) Adhesive tray/holder.

b) _____

c) _____

d) _____

e) _____

f) _____

g) _____

h) _____

i) _____

j) _____

k) _____

l) _____

m) _____

n) _____

90. ✋ **ACTIVITY**: Place the following procedural steps for False Eyelash Application in the appropriate order.

Step	Procedure
_____	Apply a thin layer of lash adhesive to the false eyelash strip and allow a few seconds for it to set.
_____	Lightly apply mascara to the tips to minimize separation between the false and natural lashes.
_____	Brush the client's eyelashes to make sure they are clean and free of debris. Curl eyelashes with an eyelash curler before applying artificial lashes.
_____	Align the strip with the client's lash line, starting at the outer edge of the eye. Use an orange stick (wooden pusher) or the rounded edge of your tweezers to slide the strip right up to the base of the lashes.
_____	Use tweezers to remove lashes from the package. Measure strip lashes by lightly placing them along the client's lash line. Adjust the length by trimming the outer edges of each strip (band).

How to Use Special-Occasion Makeup

91. Outline the procedure for creating striking contour eyes.

a) _____

_____

b) _____

_____

c) _____

_____

d) _____

_____

e) _____

_____

f) _____

_____

g) _____

_____

92. List the steps to creating dramatic smoky eyes.

a) _____

_____

b) _____

_____

c) _____

_____

_____

_____

d) _____

_____

e) _____

_____

f) _____

_____

g) _____

_____

93. List some tips for creating a special occasion look for the cheeks.

a) _____

_____

b) _____

_____

c) _____

_____

d) _____

_____

94. List some tips for creating a special occasion look for lips.

a) _____

_____

b) _____

_____

c) _____

_____

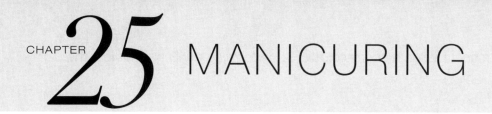

CHAPTER 25 MANICURING

Date: _____

Rating: _____

Text Pages: 848–897

why study MANICURING?

1. In your own words, explain why cosmetologists should study and thoroughly understand manicuring.

_____

_____

_____

_____

_____

_____

_____

_____

_____

_____

Adhere to State and Government Regulations

2. The list of services cosmetologists are legally allowed to perform in their specialties in their states is known as the _____.

3. A scope of practice may or may not state the services cosmetologists cannot legally perform.

   _____ True   _____ False

Rationale:

4. If damages to a client occur while a cosmetologist is performing an illegal service, the cosmetologist is not liable.

_____ True   _____ False

Rationale:

5. The Occupational Safety and Health Administration (OSHA) Hazard Communication Standard requires salon ventilation where chemical services are performed as well as proper _____.

Work with Nail Technology Tools

6. Professional cosmetologists must learn to work with the tools required for nail services and know all _____, _____, and _____ procedures as defined in your state's regulations.

7. Name the four types of nail technology tools cosmetologists will incorporate into their services.

1) _____

2) _____

3) _____

4) _____

8. _____ includes all permanent tools that are not implements that are used to perform nail services.

9. List the equipment needed to perform nail services.

a) _____

b) _____

c) _____

d) _____

e) _____

f) _____

g) _____

h) _____

i) _____

j) _____

k) _____

l) _____

m) _____

n) _____

o) _____

p) _____

10. A _____ can vary in length, but it is usually 36 inches (91.4 centimeters) to 48 inches (121.9 centimeters) long.

11. The adjustable lamp attached to a manicure table should use a 40- to 60-watt incandescent or fluorescent bulb.

_____ True   _____ False

Rationale:

12. The cosmetologist's chair should be selected for what features?

_____

_____

13. How is the finger bowl used in nail service?

_____

_____

14. UVA and LED lamps cure or harden products that contain _____, which are designed to be sensitive to the UVA wavelength the bulbs emit.

15. The warmth of electric hand/foot mitts is designed to

_____,

_____, and

_____.

16. _____, a petroleum by-product, has excellent sealing properties to hold moisture in the skin.

17. Special heating units melt solid paraffin wax into a gel-like liquid and maintain it at a temperature generally between _____ and _____ degrees Fahrenheit.

18. Fans and open windows are excellent substitutes for proper ventilation systems.

_____ True   _____ False

Rationale:

19. _____ or _____ implements are generally stainless steel because they must be properly cleaned and disinfected after use on one client and prior to use on another.

20. _____ or _____ implements cannot be reused because they cannot be cleaned and disinfected; they must be thrown away after a single use.

21. Match each of the following implements or materials with its use in nail care.

_____ Wooden pushers

_____ Metal pushers

_____ Nail brushes

_____ Nail nippers

_____ Tweezers

_____ Nail clippers

_____ Plastic or metal spatulas

_____ Two- or three-way buffers

_____ Product application brushes

a) Trim away dead skin around the nails

b) Shorten the free edge quickly and efficiently

c) Remove products from containers

d) Remove cuticle tissue from the nail plate or clean under the free edge of the nail

e) Scrub the implements clean before disinfection

f) Lift small bits of debris from the nail plate and remove implements from disinfectant solution

g) Apply nail oils, nail polish, or nail treatments to client's nails

h) Create a beautiful shine on nails

i) Gently scrape cuticle tissue from the natural nail plate

22. **ACTIVITY**: Label all the implements and materials depicted below and state their use.

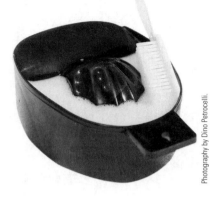

Photography by Dino Petrocelli.

_____

_____

_____

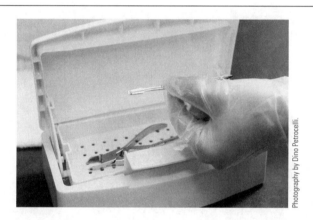

Photography by Dino Petrocelli.

_____

_____

_____

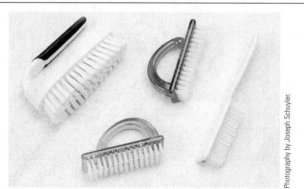

Photography by Joseph Schuyler.

_____

_____

_____

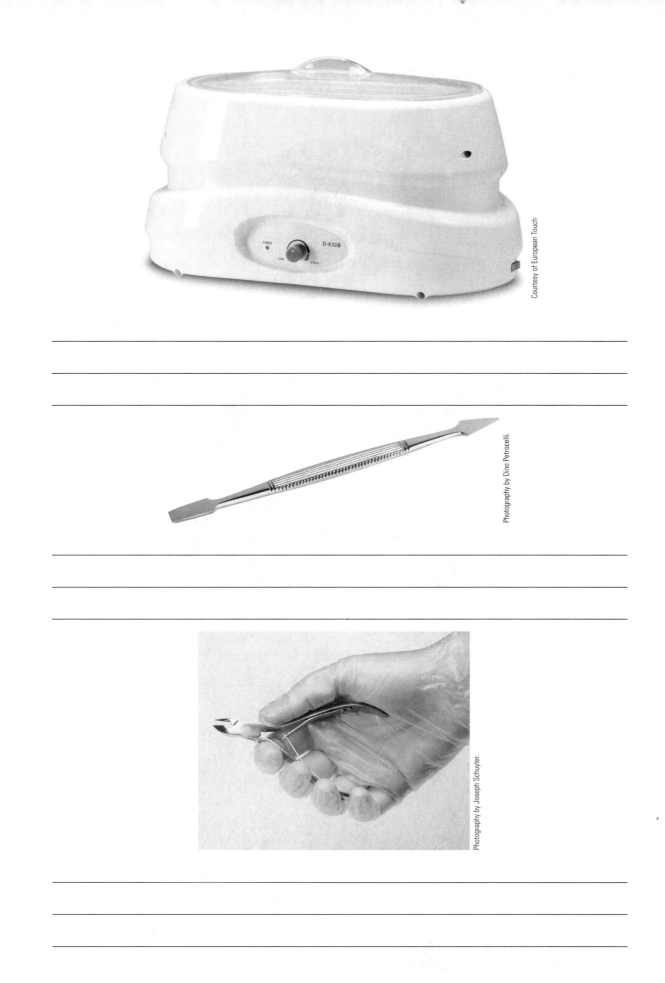

Courtesy of European Touch

Photography by Dino Petrocelli.

Photography by Joseph Schuyler.

23. Lower-grit abrasives, which are less than _____ grit, are aggressive, while fine-grit abrasives, in the category of _____ and higher grits, are designed for buffing, polishing, and removing very fine scratches.

24. If a single client receives both a manicure and a pedicure, the cosmetologist needs only one set of gloves.

    _____ True   _____ False

    Rationale:

25. Why should a cosmetologist exercise caution when buffing the nail plate during a basic manicure?

    _____

    _____

    _____

26. Why are liquid soaps preferred professional cosmetic products?

    _____

    _____

    _____

27. _____ are used to dissolve and remove nail polish.

28. _____ polish remover works more quickly and is a better solvent than _____ based removers, which are preferred when removing nail polish from nail enhancements.

29. What are nail creams, lotions, and oils designed to do?

    _____

    _____

    _____

    _____

30. Discuss the use of cuticle removers in nail care.

_____

_____

_____

_____

31. Excessive exposure of the eponychium to cuticle removers can cause _____

_____.

32. What is nail bleach?

_____

_____

_____

_____

33. Discuss what the cosmetologist should do when performing a basic manicure on a client with yellow nails.

_____

_____

_____

_____

_____

_____

34. What are the alternate names for the colored coatings applied to the natural nail plate?

a) _____

b) _____

c) _____

d) _____

35. _____ is a generic term describing any type of solvent-based colored film applied to the nail plate for the purpose of adding color or special visual effects.

36. Why is it important to use base coats on nail enhancements?

_____

_____

37. Nail hardeners can be applied before the base coat or after as top coat.

_____ True   _____ False

Rationale:

38. List some basic types of nail hardeners.

a) _____

b) _____

c) _____

39. Explain the use of top coats in cosmetology.

_____

_____

_____

_____

_____

40. Contrast hand creams and lotions.

_____

_____

_____

_____

_____

41. UVA is known to cause age spots, also called _____, on the backs of the hands and damage to the DNA of skin cells.

Learn the Necessary Components
to Perform the Basic Manicure

42. Before leaving school, cosmetology students should work to get the basic manicure procedure to _____ minutes at the most, including polishing.

43. Outline the process for cleaning and disinfecting implements as part of the pre-service procedure.

_____

_____

_____

_____

_____

_____

_____

_____

_____

_____

_____

_____

_____

_____

44. List the steps in the post-service procedure.

a) _____

b) _____

c) _____

45. During the nail consultation, what should the cosmetologist evaluate the nails for?

a) _____

b) _____

c) _____

46. Explain the last step of the manicure consultation.

_____

_____

_____

_____

47. List the five basic nail shapes women most often prefer.

1) _____

2) _____

3) _____

4) _____

5) _____

48. List the four coats of a successful nail polish application.

1) _____

2) _____

3) _____

4) _____

49. List the steps for applying colored nail polish.

a) _____

_____

_____

_____

_____

b) _____

_____

_____

_____

c) _____

_____

_____

_____

_____

d) _____

_____

_____

_____

_____

e) _____

_____

_____

_____

_____

f) _____

_____

_____

_____

_____

g) _____

_____

_____

_____

_____

50. Building nail polish layer by layer improves adhesion and staying power.

_____ True   _____ False

Rationale:

How to Cater to a Man's Manicure Service

51. A man's manicure is executed using the same basic manicure procedure you would perform on a woman, though you omit the _____

    _____.

52. Square nails are the most common choice for male clients.

_____ True   _____ False

Rationale:

53. Why must the cosmetologist prepare a man's nails for polish carefully?

    _____

    _____

    _____

    _____

    _____

54. Explain how a salon can effectively market nail services to men.

    _____

    _____

    _____

    _____

    _____

55. Explain how to make men feel more comfortable in the salon during nail care services.

_____

_____

_____

_____

_____

Complete a Hand and Arm Massage

56. _____ is the manipulation of the soft tissues of the body.

57. The cosmetologist should always have one hand on the client's arm or hand during massage movements and the transitions between them.

_____ True   _____ False

Rationale:

58. Identify the massage movements that are usually combined to complete a massage.

a) _____

b) _____

c) _____

d) _____

e) _____

59. _____ is a succession of strokes in which the hands glide over an area of the body with varying degrees of pressure or contact.

60. Hand and/or arm massage is contraindicated for clients with _____
_____.

61. What action is essential after a massage?

_____

_____

62. Explain how to perform effleurage on the arm as part of the hand and arm massage procedure.

_____

_____

_____

_____

_____

_____

_____

_____

_____

63. What does the accompanying figure depict?

_____

_____

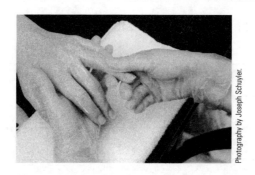

Photography by Joseph Schuyler.

State the Differences Between Spa Manicures and Basic Manicures

64. Spa manicures require more advanced techniques than basic manicures.

_____ True   _____ False

Rationale:

65. All spa manicures include some form of _____ for not only polishing and smoothing the skin, but also for enhancing penetration of professional products.

66. Identify the additional techniques that may be incorporated into a spa manicure.

a) _____

b) _____

c) _____

Indicate Why Aromatherapy is Used During a Nail Service

67. The practice of _____ involves the use of highly concentrated essential oils that are extracted using various forms of distillation from seeds, bark, roots, leaves, wood, and/or resin of plants.

Summarize the Benefits of Paraffin Wax Treatments

68. Explain the basic intent of paraffin wax treatments.

_____

_____

_____

_____

_____

69. Name the two advantages of performing a paraffin wax treatment before beginning a manicure.

1) _____

_____

2) _____

_____

Outline Nail Art Options for Clients

70. Polish is most often used to create nail art looks such as French manicures, color fades, _____, or _____.

71. A tool with a solid handle with a rounded ball tip on each end that can range in size is known as a _____ .

Only the Beginning

72. During your time in school, it is important that you learn the basic procedures of nail technology, as well as the importance of _____, _____, and other skills necessary for ensuring client safety and enjoyment during nail procedures.

CHAPTER 26 PEDICURING

Date: _____

Rating: _____

Text Pages: 898–925

1. A(n) _____ is a cosmetic service performed on the feet by a licensed cosmetologist or nail technician, can include exfoliating the skin, _____, and trimming, shaping, and polishing the toenails.

2. Pedicures are merely manicures on the feet.

   _____ True   _____ False

Rationale:

3. Pedicures present more potential for damage to clients than do manicures.

   _____ True   _____ False

Rationale:

4. List some reasons why pedicures are beneficial.

   a) _____

   b) _____

   c) _____

   d) _____

why study PEDICURING?

5. In your own words, explain why cosmetologists should study and thoroughly understand pedicuring.

_____

_____

_____

_____

_____

Learn the Tools and Materials Used During Pedicures

6. Name the four types of nail technology tools the cosmetologist will use during the pedicure service.

1) _____

2) _____

3) _____

4) _____

7. Some permanent equipment for performing pedicures differs from that used for standard manicures.

_____ True   _____ False

Rationale:

8. Which of the following pieces of pedicure equipment is considered optional?

_____ a) Paraffin bath   _____ c) Pedicure cart

_____ b) Pedicure footrest   _____ d) Pedicure foot bath

9. Give four examples of pedicure foot baths in increasing order of sophistication.

1) _____

_____

_____

_____

2) _____

_____

_____

_____

_____

3) _____

_____

_____

_____

_____

4) _____

_____

_____

_____

10. Contrast electric foot mitts with terry cloth mitts.

_____

_____

_____

_____

_____

_____

_____

_____

11. List some pedicure-specific implements.

a) _____

b) _____

c) _____

d) _____

e) _____

f) _____

12. Describe how to use a nail rasp during the basic pedicure procedure.

_____

_____

_____

_____

13. Identify the materials unique to pedicuring, as well as their uses.

a) _____

_____

b) _____

_____

14. Name the professional products that are unique to pedicuring.

a) _____

b) _____

c) _____

d) _____

e) _____

15. _____ are products that are put into the water in the pedicure bath to soften the skin on the feet during the soak time.

16. Exfoliating scrubs are usually _____ -based lotions that contain a(n) _____ as the exfoliating agent.

17. What are some popular ingredients in masks?

_____

_____

18. Callus softeners are applied directly to the client's calluses and are left on for a short period of time, according to the manufacturer's directions.

_____ True   _____ False

Rationale:

Know All About Pedicures

19. Give some guidelines for choosing pedicure products.

a) _____

_____

_____

b) _____

_____

_____

c) _____

_____

_____

20. Discuss the benefit of short pedicure services.

_____

_____

_____

_____

_____

21. Why should female clients avoid shaving their legs for the 48 hours preceding a pedicure?

_____

_____

_____

_____

22. If the client's feet are in bad shape, you should work as long as necessary to get them in optimal condition in only one service.

_____ True   _____ False

Rationale:

23. Discuss the concept of the series pedicure, and give an example.

_____

_____

_____

24. List the steps below for a basic pedicure. The first two steps have been listed to help you get started.

a) Check the temperature of the pedicure bath for safety. Put on a pair of clean gloves, place the client's feet in the bath, and make sure he or she is comfortable with the water temperature. Allow the feet to soak for 5 to 10 minutes to soften and clean the feet before beginning the pedicure.

b) Lift the client's foot you will be working with first from the bath. Using the towels on the footrest, on the pedicure cart, or on your lap, wrap the first towel around the foot and dry it thoroughly. Make sure you dry between the toes. If you are using a basin or portable bath, place the foot on the footrest or on a towel you have placed on your lap.

c) _____

_____

_____

_____

_____

d) _____

_____

_____

_____

_____

e) _____

_____

_____

_____

f) _____

_____

_____

_____

g) _____

_____

_____

_____

h) _____

_____

_____

_____

i) _____

_____

_____

_____

j) _____

_____

_____

_____

k) _____

_____

_____

_____

_____

l) _____

_____

_____

_____

_____

m) _____

_____

_____

_____

_____

n) _____

_____

_____

_____

_____

o) _____

_____

_____

_____

_____

p) _____

_____

_____

_____

q) _____

_____

_____

_____

_____

r) _____

_____

_____

_____

_____

s) _____

_____

_____

_____

_____

25. The basic pedicure is the basis for all other pedicure services. For example, in the basic pedicure, the massage is performed on the foot only, while in the upgrade to a _____, the massage is performed on the foot and the lower leg _____.

26. Older people need less regular foot care than younger people.

_____ True   _____ False

Rationale:

27. For an elderly client receiving pedicure services, a microscopic opening, or _____, can be fatal.

28. What is another great way to upgrade your pedicure service and price?

_____

29. According to client salon surveys, _____ is the most enjoyed aspect of any nail service.

30. Massage given during manicures and pedicures focuses on therapy.

_____ True   _____ False

Rationale:

31. During the client consultation, you should acknowledge and discuss any medical condition your client listed that may be _____ for a foot and/or leg massage.

32. Foot and/or leg massage is contraindicated for clients with severe,

_____

33. Describe how to grasp the foot when performing a pedicure.

_____

_____

34. Explain how to use lotion or oil during a foot and leg massage.

_____

_____

_____

_____

_____

_____

_____

35. The bottom of the foot is the only place a friction movement is performed in pedicure services.

_____ True   _____ False

Rationale:

36. What is the role of feathering in foot and leg massage?

_____

_____

_____

37. Describe the subject of the accompanying figure.

_____

_____

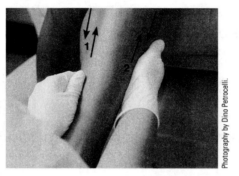

Photography by Dino Petrocelli.

38. 🖐 ACTIVITY: Place the following procedural steps for a Foot and Leg Massage in the appropriate order.

Step   **Procedure**

_____   Place one hand on top of the foot, cupping it, and make a fist with the other hand. The hand on top of the foot will press the foot toward you while your other hand twists into the instep of the foot (friction movement). This helps stimulate the blood flow and provides relaxation. Repeat three to five times.

_____   End the massage with a feathering technique to provide a signal for experienced clients that the massage is ending. Finish by placing both of the client's feet onto the footrest, and firmly press the tops of the feet three times slowly for one or two seconds each, and then allow the client to relax a minute or two before moving to the next step of the procedure.

_____   Put on a fresh pair of gloves and rest the client's heel on a footrest or stool and suggest that your client relax. Grasp the leg gently above the ankle and use your other hand to hold the foot just beneath the toes; rotate the entire foot in a circular motion.

_____   Place the foot on the footrest or stabilize it on your lap, then gently grasp the client's leg from behind the ankle with one hand. Perform effleurage movements from the ankle to below the knee on the front of the leg with the other hand. Move up the leg and then lightly return to the original location. Perform five to seven repetitions, then move to the sides of the leg and perform an additional five to seven repetitions.

_____ Hold the tip of the toe, starting with the little toe, and make a figure eight with each toe. Repeat three to five times on each toe and then move to the next. After the last movement on each toe, gently squeeze the tip of each once, and then move on to the next toe.

_____ While holding the ankle, place the palm of your free hand on top of the foot behind the toes. Slide the palm up to the ankle area with gentle pressure and then return to starting position. Repeat three to five times in the middle, then on the sides of the top of the foot.

_____ Perform the same thumb movement on the surface of the heels, rotating your thumbs in opposite directions. Repeat three to five times.

_____ Return your hands to the position described in step 4 and repeat steps 3 and 4. Repeat all movements on each foot as many times as you wish, adding other movements that you like to perform, and then move to the other leg/ foot.

_____ Slide to the back of the legs and perform effleurage movements up the back of the leg. Stroke up the leg, then, with less pressure, return to the original location; perform five to seven times.

_____ Repeat the same motions of step 3 with the opposite hand and thumb. The base of the thumbs to the pads of the fingers should be in contact with the skin throughout the movement. Alternate this massage step with each hand and thumb and repeat several times.

_____ Start with the little toe, placing the thumb on the top of the toe and curl the index finger underneath the toe. (Your palm is facing up.) Push the fingers and thumb in that position back to the base of the toe, then rotate the thumb and finger in a circular, effleurage movement until the index finger is arched over the top of the toe, and the thumb is underneath. Pull the toe with index finger and thumb outward, away from the foot.

_____ Once the massage of both feet is completed, you may move on in the pedicure procedure. If you are performing a luxury pedicure, do not perform the feather off movement; slide your hands to the leg and move on to the leg massage after step 9.

_____ Never losing contact with the skin, slide your hands so that the thumbs are on the plantar side of the foot while the fingers are gently holding the dorsal side of the foot, like holding a sandwich. Move one thumb in a firm circular movement, moving from one side of the foot, across, above the heel, up the medial side (center side) of the foot to below the toes, across the ball of the foot and back down to the other side of the foot (distal side) to the original position.

39. Give a brief overview of reflexology.

_____

_____

_____

_____

40. List the two reasons professional, hands-on training is essential in reflexology.

    1) _____

    _____

    2) _____

    _____

41. When giving a pedicure, pay attention to your body's positioning and make sure you are working _____.

Properly Clean and Disinfect Foot Spas

42. The disinfecting procedures for manicuring and pedicuring have been developed by the _____, a group of nail-care company representatives, and the _____, a group of professional nail technicians, for cleaning and disinfecting all types of pedicure equipment.

CHAPTER 27 NAIL TIPS & WRAPS

Date: _____

Rating: _____

Text Pages: 926–949

why study NAIL TIPS & WRAPS?

1. In your own words, explain why cosmetologists should study and thoroughly understand nail tips and nail wraps.

_____

_____

_____

_____

_____

_____

_____

_____

_____

_____

Learn All You Need to Know About Nail Tips

2. Nail tips are plastic, pre-molded nails shaped from a tough polymer made from _____ plastic.

3. Tips are combined with a(n) _____, a layer of any kind of nail enhancement product that is applied over the natural nail and tip application for added strength.

4. In addition to basic materials, what implements are needed on the manicuring table?

a) _____

b) _____

c) _____

d) _____

e) _____

f) _____

5. Fingernail clippers should be used to cut tips.

_____ True   _____ False

Rationale:

6. Define the roles of the well and the position stop.

_____

_____

_____

7. The bonding agent used to secure the nail tip to the natural nail is called the

_____.

8. Cosmetologists and their clients should always wear eye protection when using and handling nail tip adhesives.

_____ True   _____ False

Rationale:

9. Explain the proper way to apply adhesive during nail tip application.

_____

_____

Explore the Uses of Nail Wraps

10. Any method of securing a layer of fabric or paper on and around the nail tip to ensure its strength and durability is called a(n) _____.

11. Wrap resins are made from _____, a specialized acrylic monomer that has excellent adhesion to the natural nail plate and polymerizes in seconds.

12. Fabric wraps are the most popular type of nail wrap because of their durability.

    _____ True   _____ False

Rationale:

13. Compare silk wraps and linen wraps.

    _____

    _____

    _____

    _____

    _____

    _____

    _____

14. Why are paper wraps considered a temporary service?

    _____

    _____

    _____

    _____

15. A(n) _____, also known as an activator, acts as the dryer that speeds the hardening process of the wrap resin or adhesive overlay.

16. Name the implements and materials needed for nail wrap application.

a) _____

b) _____

c) _____

d) _____

e) _____

f) _____

g) _____

h) _____

17. (W) **ACTIVITY:** Practice nail tip and wrap applications on your own non-dominant hand. Select tips that fit each of the five fingers on your non-dominant hand and apply them according to the procedure outlined in this chapter. Then apply different wraps on the nails using at least one silk wrap, one paper wrap, one linen wrap, and one fiberglass wrap. After successful completion of the wraps, apply polish to the nails. Perform a thorough analysis of each wrap style. Consider the ease of application and the smoothness of the polish based on your application. Make a recommendation based on your experiment as to which wrap method you would recommend for your client and why. State your findings below.

_____

_____

_____

_____

_____

Carry Out Nail Wrap Maintenance, Repair, and Removal

18. What two goals does nail maintenance accomplish?

1) _____

_____

2) _____

_____

19. Outline the steps to two-week fabric wrap maintenance. The first two steps have been provided to help you get started.

a) Use a non-acetone polish remover to remove existing nail polish and to avoid damaging nail wraps. Acetone will break down the wrap resin too quickly.

b) Clean the natural nails.

c) _____

_____

_____

d) _____

_____

_____

e) _____

_____

_____

f) _____

_____

_____

g) _____

_____

_____

h) _____

_____

_____

i) _____

_____

_____

j) _____

_____

_____

k) _____

_____

_____

l) _____

_____

_____

m) _____

_____

_____

n) _____

_____

_____

20. A _____ is a piece of fabric cut to ⅛-inch (3.12 mm) in length and applied to strengthen a weak point in the nail.

21. A _____ is a piece of fabric cut to completely cover a crack or break in the nail.

22. Explain how to buff the nail during the procedure for four-week fabric wrap maintenance.

_____

_____

_____

_____

_____

_____

23. Discuss the proper procedure for removing fabric nail wraps.

_____

_____

_____

_____

_____

24. Detail the steps in nail tip removal. The first step is listed to help you get started.

a) Start by applying a thick lotion or barrier cream to the hands and cuticle. This will help protect the surrounding skin prior to soaking in acetone or product remover.

b) _____

_____

_____

_____

c) _____

_____

_____

_____

d) _____

_____

_____

_____

e) _____

_____

_____

_____

Date: _____

Rating: _____

Text Pages: 950–985

why study MONOMER LIQUID & POLYMER POWDER NAIL ENHANCEMENTS?

1. In your own words, explain why cosmetologists should study and thoroughly understand monomer liquid and polymer powder nail enhancements.

_____

_____

_____

_____

_____

_____

_____

_____

Convey the Chemistry of Monomer Liquid and Polymer Powder Nail Enhancements

2. Monomer liquid and polymer powder nail enhancements, also known as _____, are created by combining a chemical known as _____ liquid mixed, with _____ powder, to form a nail enhancement.

3. The ingredients in two-part monomer liquid and polymer powder nail enhancement systems belong to a branch of the acrylic family called _____.

4. _____ means one and _____ stands for units, so a _____ is one unit called a molecule. _____ means many, so _____ means a substance formed by combining many small molecules into very long, chain-like structures.

5. List the four basic ways monomer liquid and polymer powder products can be applied.

   1) _____

   2) _____

   3) _____

   4) _____

6. In addition to the basic materials on the manicuring table, list the supplies needed for the procedure for one-color monomer liquid and polymer powder nail enhancements over nail tips or natural nails.

   a) _____

   b) _____

   c) _____

   d) _____

   e) _____

   f) _____

   g) _____

   h) _____

7. A _____ brush is the best brush to use for applying monomer liquid and polymer powder nail enhancements.

8. List the three versions of monomer liquid usually used in the beauty industry.

   1) _____

   2) _____

   3) _____

9. Describe what occurs during the chemical reaction called polymerization.

   _____

   _____

   _____

10. _____, additives designed to speed up chemical reactions, are added to monomer liquid and used to control the set or curing time. _____, found in polymer powder, when activated by a catalyst, will spring into action and cause monomer molecules to permanently link together into long polymer chains.

11. Explain why it is important to use the polymer powder designed for a specific monomer liquid.

_____

_____

_____

Specify the Supplies Required for Monomer Liquid and Polymer Powder Nail Enhancements

12. The amount of monomer liquid and polymer powder used to create a bead is called the

_____.

13. Compare dry, wet, and medium mix ratios.

_____

_____

_____

_____

14. In general, medium beads are the ideal mix ratio for working with monomer liquids and polymer powders.

_____ True   _____ False

Rationale:

15. The color of polymer powder depends on the nail enhancement method being used.

_____ True   _____ False

Rationale:

16. Explain the use of nail dehydrators.

_____

_____

17. Acid-based nail primers are used most often today.

_____ True   _____ False

Rationale:

18. Outline the procedure for using nonacid and acid-free nail primers.

_____

_____

_____

_____

_____

_____

_____

_____

_____

_____

19. High-quality hand sanitizers can replace hand washing in many cases.

_____ True   _____ False

Rationale:

20. Choose a _____-grit abrasive for smoothing the surface and a _____-grit abrasive for finish filing, refining, and buffing.

21. _____ are placed under the free edge of the natural nail and used as a guide to extend nail enhancements beyond the fingertips for additional length.

22. Describe the appropriate containers for monomer liquid and polymer powder.

_____

_____

_____

_____

_____

_____

23. Explain why brushes of natural kolinsky, sable, or a blend of both are the best for monomer liquid and polymer powder nail enhancements.

_____

_____

_____

24. Dust masks are worn to provide vapor protection.

_____ True   _____ False

Rationale:

25. For many salon-related applications, gloves made of nitrile polymer powder work best.

_____ True   _____ False

Rationale:

26. Explain how to store monomer liquid and polymer powder products.

_____

_____

_____

27. To dispose of small amounts of monomer liquid, mix them with small amounts of the powder designed to cure them.

_____ True   _____ False

Rationale:

Complete Monomer Liquid and Polymer Powder Nail Enhancement Maintenance, Crack Repair, and Removal

28. What is the preferred maintenance schedule for monomer liquid and polymer powder nail enhancements?

_____

_____

29. List the steps in the one-color monomer liquid and polymer powder maintenance procedure. A few steps are provided to help you get started.

a) Remove the existing polish or gel sealant, then use a pusher to gently push back the eponychium and carefully remove cuticle tissue from the nail plate.

b) Using a medium-coarse abrasive (150- to 180-grit) flat against the existing product, carefully smooth down the ledge until it is flush with the new growth of nail plate. Smooth out any areas of product that may be lifting or forming pockets. Be careful not to damage the natural nail plate with your abrasive.

c) _____

_____

_____

d) _____

_____

_____

e) _____

_____

_____

f) Apply nail dehydrator to all nails.

g) _____

_____

_____

h) _____

_____

_____

i) _____

_____

_____

j) _____

_____

_____

_____

k) _____

_____

_____

l) _____

_____

_____

m) _____

_____

_____

n) _____

_____

_____

o) _____

_____

p) _____

_____

_____

_____

q) _____

_____

_____

r) Polish nail enhancements depending on your client's preferences.

30. In an abbreviated manner, list below the steps for crack repair for monomer liquid and polymer powder nail enhancements. The first two steps have been listed to get you started.

a) Remove existing polish or gel sealant and push back the eponychium.

b) Gently file the nail surface with a medium/fine abrasive. Remove the nail dust with a clean, dry nail brush.

c) _____

_____

d) _____

_____

e) _____

_____

f) _____

_____

g) _____

_____

h) _____

_____

i) _____

_____

j) _____

_____

k) _____

_____

l) _____

_____

m) _____

_____

n) _____

_____

o) _____

_____

p) _____

_____

31. The _____, also known as arch, is the area of the nail that has the most strength.

32. The stress area is the area on the side of the nail plate that grows free of its attachment to the nail fold and where the extension leaves the natural nail.

_____ True   _____ False

Rationale:

33. Discuss the nail extension underside.

_____

_____

_____

_____

_____

_____

34. In an abbreviated manner, list the steps in the procedure for monomer liquid and polymer powder nail enhancement removal. The first step has been listed to help you get started.

a) Have client wash hands; remove existing polish; apply thick lotion to hands and cuticle.

b) _____

_____

_____

_____

c) _____

_____

_____

_____

d) _____

_____

_____

_____

e) _____

_____

_____

_____

f) _____

_____

_____

_____

g) _____

_____

_____

_____

h) _____

_____

_____

i) _____

_____

_____

Decsribe Odorless Monomer Liquid and Polymer Powder Products

35. Odorless monomer liquid and polymer powder products have little odor.

_____ True   _____ False

Rationale:

36. Define the inhibition layer of odorless products, and explain how to remove it.

_____

_____

_____

_____

Utilize Colored Polymer Powder Products

37. Polymer powders are now available in a wide range of colors that mimic almost every shade available in nail polish.

_____ True   _____ False

Rationale:

Create Monomer Liquid and Polymer Powder Nail Art

38. Monomer liquid and polymer powder can be used in a variety of ways to create unique _____.

39. Three dimensional, or 3-D nail art, describes any art that _____ from the nail. When applying 3-D art over nail polish, the polish should be dried for at least _____ minutes before applying the art.

40. Inlaid designs, designs inside a nail enhancement, are created when nail art _____ of product while the nail enhancement is being formed.

41. ⓦ **ACTIVITY:** Conduct an Internet search for "acrylic fingernails," and print at least a dozen images of different monomer liquid and polymer powder fingernails with nail art. Attempt to identify and list the methods and procedures used to create the end result of each image. With your instructor's permission, attempt to duplicate the look of one image either on a mannequin hand or finger, a fellow student, or a model.

_____

_____

_____

29 LIGHT CURED GELS

Date: _____

Rating: _____

Text Pages: 986–1021

1. A _____ is a type of nail enhancement product that hardens when exposed to a UV and LED light source.

why study LIGHT CURED GELS?

2. In your own words, explain why cosmetologists should study and thoroughly understand light cured gels.

_____

_____

_____

_____

_____

_____

_____

Comprehend the Chemistry of Light Cured Gels

3. Nail enhancements based on light curing are very similar to methacrylates.

_____ True   _____ False

Rationale:

4. Although most light cured gels are made from _____, new light cured gel technologies have been developed that use methacrylates.

5. Like wraps and monomer liquid and polymer powder nail enhancements, light cured gels can also contain _____ liquids, but they rely mostly on a related form called a(n) _____.

6. The term _____ means which of the following?

   _____ a) One   _____ c) Few

   _____ b) Many   _____ d) Outside

7. Explain the concept of an oligomer.

   _____

   _____

   _____

8. Oligomers are between solid and liquid.

   _____ True   _____ False

Rationale:

9. Traditionally, light cured gels rely on a special type of acrylate called a(n) _____ acrylate, while newer light cured gel systems use

   _____.

10. The term _____ refers to the type of starting material that is used to create the most common light cured gel resins.

11. The chemical family of urethanes is known for high abrasion resistance and durability.

    _____ True   _____ False

Rationale:

12. A chemical called a _____ initiates the polymerization reaction.

13. Light cured gel systems employ multiple resin compounds that are cured to a solid material when exposed to a UV or LED light source.

_____ True   _____ False

Rationale:

14. After the nail plate is properly prepared, each layer of product applied to the natural nail, nail tip, or form requires exposure to a UV or LED light to _____ or harden.

Describe Light Cured Gels

15. Identify the four different types of UV gels.

1) _____

2) _____

3) _____

4) _____

16. Describe the one-color method for applying light cured gels.

_____

_____

_____

_____

17. Describe the two-color method for applying light cured gels.

_____

_____

_____

_____

18. List the implements and materials needed for the one-color method for applying UV or LED gel on tips or natural nails finishing with UV or LED gel polish.

a) _____

b) _____

c) _____

d) _____

e) _____

f) _____

g) _____

h) _____

i) _____

j) _____

19. Explain how to apply the first layer of UV or LED gel to the fingernail surface using the one-color method.

_____

_____

_____

_____

20. Complete the two-color method for applying UV or LED gel to tips or natural nails by filling in the missing steps.

a) Clean the nails, and remove existing polish.

b) Apply cuticle remover to the nail plate, if needed. Gently push back the eponychium, and remove cuticle tissue from the nail plate.

c) _____

_____

_____

d) Remove the dust from the nail surfaces.

e) Use a cleanser and dehydrator per the manufacturer's recommendation to remove any oils and debris from the fingernail. This increases the adhesive properties of the gel.

f) _____

_____

_____

g) Cure bonding gel, if required, following the manufacturer's directions.

h) _____

_____

_____

_____

_____

i) Using a lint-free nail wipe, pinch the bristles of the brush in the nail wipe to pull off excess gel. Do not use solvents to clean the bristles.

j) _____

_____

_____

_____

k) _____

_____

l) If the white gel does not have the same brightness and consistency on all fingers, repeat steps h through k.

m) Gently float a pink-tinted gel onto the fingernail surface, including the free edge. Leave a 3/16-inch (4.76 mm) gap around the cuticle and the sidewall area of the fingernail. Keep the gel from touching the cuticle, eponychium, or sidewalls.

n) _____

_____

o) Repeat steps m and n on the left hand, and then repeat the steps for both thumbs.

p) _____

_____

_____

_____

q) _____

_____

r) Repeat steps p and q on the left hand, and then repeat the same steps for both thumbs.

s) Another layer of the UV or LED gel will add thickness to the enhancement if it is desired. Cure the nails.

t) _____

_____

u) Contour the nails with a medium/fine-grit abrasive (180- or 240-grit).

v) Remove the dust with a nylon brush. Evaluate the work you just completed and make any necessary adjustments.

w) _____

_____

x) Remove the inhibition layer, if required.

y) Apply and rub nail oil into the surrounding skin, massaging briefly to speed up penetration.

z) _____

_____

_____

_____

aa) Apply hand cream and massage the hand and arms. Thoroughly clean each nail of lotion.

21. _____ are used to increase adhesion to the natural nail plate, similar to a monomer liquid and polymer powder primer.

22. A bonding product that is not cured in a UV or LED lamp is less effective than one cured in a UV or LED lamp.

_____ True   _____ False

Rationale:

23. Which of the following type of gel is used to enhance the thickness of the overlay while providing a smoother surface?

_____ a) Gel polish   _____ c) Glossing gel

_____ b) Pigmented gel   _____ d) Self-leveling gel

24. _____ gels are very helpful when repairing a break or crack in a client's enhancement.

25. ⊕ **ACTIVITY:** In the chart below, compare and contrast the different types of gels by describing each and how they work.

_____

_____

Gel Type	Gel Analysis
Bonding gels	• • • • • • •
Building gels	• • • • •

Gels
containing
fiberglass

-
-
-

Self-leveling
gels

-
-
-

Pigmented
gels

-
-
-
-

Gel polish

-
-
-
-
-
-

Glossing gels	•
	•
	•
	•
	•
	•

26. A(n) _____ layer is a tacky surface left on the nail after a UV or LED gel has cured.

27. Opacity is the amount of colored pigment concentration in a gel, making it more or less difficult to see through.

_____ True   _____ False

Rationale:

Name the Supplies Required for Light Cured Gels

28. Primers and bonding gels are designed specifically to _____ of UV and LED gel to the natural nail plate.

29. When selecting nail tips for a light cured gel procedure, it is important to ensure

_____.

When to Use Light Cured Gels

30. The new light cured resign technology allows light cured gel manufacturers to create _____, _____, and _____products that will perform as well as many of the monomer liquid and polymer powder systems on the market.

31. Explain how to refine the surface contour when sculpting light cured gel using forms.

_____

_____

_____

_____

_____

32. When applying monomer liquid and polymer powder nail enhancements finished with UV or LED gel polish, explain how the gel polish top gel, sealer, finish, or glass gel is applied.

_____

_____

_____

_____

_____

Choose the Proper Light Cured Gel Technology

33. Give some guidelines for choosing the proper light cured gel.

a) If the client has flat fingernails: _____

_____

_____

b) If the client has fingernails that arch and curve: _____

_____

c) If the client returns to the salon often with broken enhancements: _____

_____

d) If a client is in search of a manicure with long-lasting polish: _____

_____

Distinguish the Difference Between Light Cured Bulbs and Lamps

34. Explain the difference between a UV bulb and a UV lamp.

_____

_____

_____

_____

35. Lamp wattage is the measure of how much electricity the bulb consumes.

_____ True   _____ False

Rationale:

36. If a gel product is exposed to ceiling or table bulbs, what may occur?

_____

_____

_____

_____

_____

37. Why is it important to use the UV lamp that was designed for the UV gel product being used?

_____

_____

_____

_____

_____

38. How often should UV bulbs be changed, depending on the frequency of use?

_____ a) Monthly　　　　　　_____ c) Two or three times annually

_____ b) Once annually　　　　_____ d) Every one to three years

39. Give some potential results of failing to regularly change UV lamps.

a) _____

b) _____

c) _____

40. The most common UV lamp on the market is a _____-watt bulb.

_____ a) four　　　　　　　_____ c) seven

_____ b) six　　　　　　　　_____ d) nine

41. The lamp has as much to do with proper curing of the UV or LED gel as the bulb.

_____ True　　　　　_____ False

Rationale:

Specify the Advantages of Light Cured Gel Polish

42. Name two advantages of UV gel polishes.

1) _____

2) _____

Relate Nail Art to Light Cured Gels

43. Inlaid art in light cured gel nails is art sandwiched between _____ layers of enhancement products.

44. With inlaid art on light cured gel nails, the surface of the nail is smooth and the nail structure is not _____.

Perform Light Cured Gel Maintenance and Removal

45. Explain how to begin a UV gel maintenance.

_____

_____

_____

_____

_____

_____

_____

_____

_____

_____

46. Hard UV and LED gels, also known as _____, cannot be removed with a solvent, such as acetone. They must be _____ to be removed.

47. Soft UV and LED gels, also known as _____, including gel polishes, are removed by soaking in acetone for approximately 5 to 15 minutes or product remover to soften them, allowing the cosmetologist to easily scrape off the loosened gel polish with a _____.

48. Outline the detailed procedure for light cured gel maintenance. A few steps are provided to help you get started.

   a) Clean the nails with soap and water, and dry hands thoroughly. Remove the existing polish.

   b) Apply cuticle remover to the nail plate if needed. Gently push back the eponychium and remove cuticle from the nail plate.

   c) _____

   _____

   d) _____

   _____

e) _____

_____

_____

f) _____

_____

_____

g) _____

_____

_____

h) Cure the bonding gel if required.

i) _____

_____

_____

j) _____

_____

_____

k) Repeat steps i and j on the client's left hand. Then repeat the same steps for both thumbs.

l) _____

_____

_____

m) _____

_____

_____

n) Remove the dust, and then clean the fingernails. If finishing with gel polish, do so now. Otherwise proceed to step o.

o) _____

_____

_____

p) _____

_____

_____

q) _____

_____

_____

r) Apply and rub nail oil into the surrounding skin and nail enhancement, massaging briefly to speed up penetration.

s) _____

_____

_____

_____

t) _____

_____

_____

_____

u) Apply nail polish, if desired.

49. List the steps for removing light cured hard gel.

a) _____

_____

_____

_____

b) _____

_____

_____

_____

c) _____

_____

_____

_____

d) _____

_____

_____

_____

50. Complete the missing steps in the procedure for removing light cured soft or soakable gel polishes.

a) _____

_____

b) Pour the soak-off solution in a finger bowl or other glass or metal container so that the level of the remover is sufficient to completely immerse the fingernails in the solution.

c) _____

_____

d) _____

_____

e) _____

_____

f) While massaging nail oil into the nail and surrounding skin, evaluate the work you just completed, and make any necessary adjustments. Have your client wash her hands and dry thoroughly. Perform an arm and hand massage before completing the service.

CHAPTER **30** PREPARING FOR LICENSURE & EMPLOYMENT

See Milady Standard Cosmetology Theory Workbook.

CHAPTER **31** ON THE JOB

See Milady Standard Cosmetology Theory Workbook.

CHAPTER **32** THE SALON BUSINESS

See Milady Standard Cosmetology Theory Workbook.

NOTES